Ground to Grow:
Alignment Cues
For
Yoga Students
And Teachers

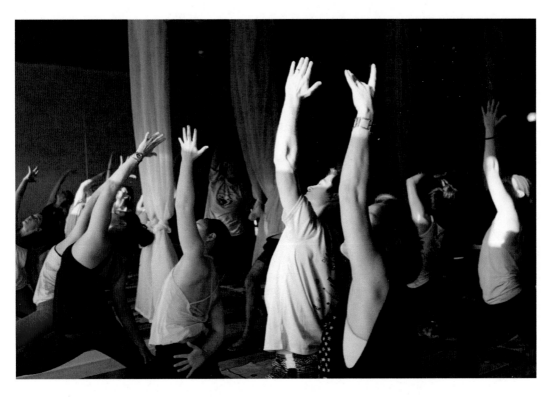

Janie Montague & Mike Luckock
Photography by Chuck Marcelo

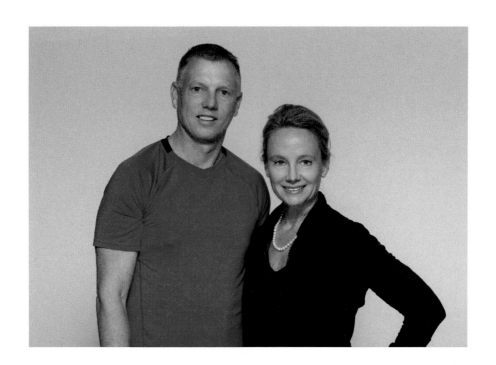

Authors

Janie Montague ERYT 200

Mike Luckock RYT 200

The information in this book is meant to supplement not replace, proper exercise training. All forms of exercise pose some inherent risks. The editors, publishers and authors advise readers to take full responsibility for their safety and to know their limits. Do not take risks beyond your level of experience, aptitude, training, and fitness. As with all exercise programs, you should get doctor's approval before beginning.

This book is conceived from a love of the practice of yoga.

It is designed as a tool to assist in the practice of finding both the words and the actions associated with the postures.

We hope this book will help you connect the foundation of the practice to the familiar and commonly used cues and terms in a yoga setting. These cues are not meant to be a script but tools teachers may bring into their classes to help connect with their students, and cues that help students effectively align the body with the approximate shape of the posture. Within the fame work of alignment and verbal cues is the ever present and paramount voice of the breath and the necessity of the student or teacher to listen and respect the feeling associated with the pose.

We have developed the book to illustrate many yoga poses. They are placed in a particular order in this book, but are not meant to be done in sequence or entirety. The poses are linked together in a Vinyasa flow class but are isolated here to teach alignment and verbal cueing. Two sided postures are cued here only one sided, ensure you balance your body by doing the opposite side.

We would like to thank the incredible students and teachers who have blessed us with their many teachings. Our gratitude is endless.

To the models in this book, thank you for your generosity, time and friendship.

The models are all yoga students or teachers and active participants in the yoga community.

Common Instructions Defined
(Cornerstones of the practice)

Breath: Ujayi Pranayama - Is the in and out flow of breath through the nose with the mouth closed. The back of the throat remains open. The breath is utilized in Vinyasa flow yoga primary to lead the movement. Almost always, the spine is extending on the inhale breath and mobilized, bending or twisting on the exhale.

Engage abdominal wall – On the inhalation breath, lift in and up from just below the navel center. Continue to lift the navel in and up even as you exhale. The contraction of the abdominal wall lifts the muscles towards centerline of the body.

Spiral the inner thighs – This muscular action is an internal or inward rotation of the quadriceps or thighs towards the centerline of the body. The thigh muscles engage and lift upwards towards the hip crease while the feet press down in standing poses.

Lengthen the tailbone – This movement is a very subtle extension of the lower spine. Lengthening is used to avoid compression of the lumbar spine. The action is initiated by tilting the pelvis into a neutral position and lifting the navel center in an up.

Keep the neck long – The action of maintaining a long neck is related to the balance of the head between the shoulders. A long neck, both side to side and front to back allows for optimal extension of the spine. The position of the chin is very helpful in keeping the front of the throat open. Lifting the chin forward and up, compresses the back of the neck and pulling the chin down and forward overextends the back of the neck; neither position are optimal. Maintaining a long, even neck, allows for the most open area for breath to flow and the head to balance.

Neutral gaze – This action is related to both the eyes and the position of the head in relation to the neck and the shoulders. The position of the eyes should keep the chin in a neutral position that will maintain the length of the neck. The eye gaze and position of the head will alleviate anything that feels like strain to the neck.

Activate/Engage- Activation or engagement of any muscle in the body is the feeling of placing awareness and attention onto the area or group of muscles, setting the muscle into motion. Sometimes motion is squeezing or contracting, other times it is lengthening and extending.

Hinge from the hips – This action of hinging or folding forward from the hip crease, below the navel center, versus folding or bending forward from the waistline is optimal for low spine health and safety. Maintain a long spine with the abdominal wall engaged.

Midline of the body – The midline of the body can be located by drawing an imaginary line from the center of the top of the head to the tailbone down the center of the spine.

Straighten - Stacking the bones without locking out the joints or hyper extending. The ligaments and muscles are supporting the stacking of the bones.

Example: A leg or arm can be in a "straightened" positioned, even if the knee or elbow is bent, as long as the bones are organized linearly, and the ligaments and muscles support the alignment and stacking of those bones.

Neutral Pelvis – Alignment of the hip bones and the pubic bones on the same plane. Ideally the pelvis is neutral when lying down or standing tall.

In this book, all instructions and cueing is directed to a person who is already in the approximate shape of the posture. The alignment cues are approximate and in the absence of fluid breath alignment has less benefit.

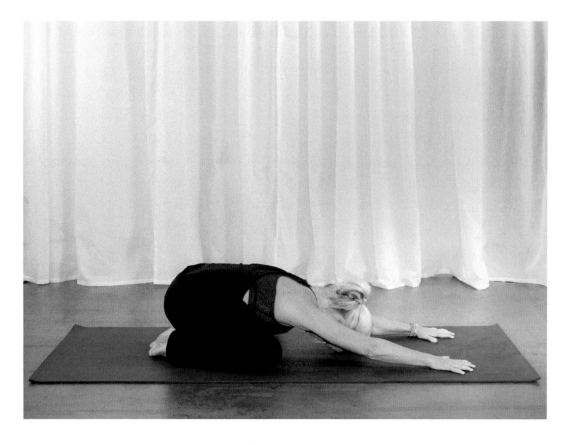

Child's (Balasana)

Press tops of feet into the ground, bring big toes to touch
Spread knees open wide or squeeze together
Lift navel center in and up to engage the abdominal wall
Drawn hips back over heels
Extend arms forward, press hands down to activate the forearms
Draw shoulder blades draw back and down the spine
Relax the forehead on the mat, roll hairline left to right
Gaze toward tip of nose or navel

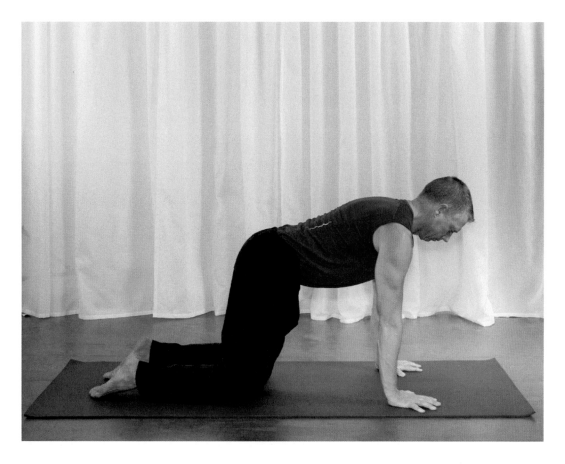

All Fours

Stack hips over knees
Spiral the thighs toward the midline of the body
Align wrist, elbows and shoulders, flatten palms
Maintain a flat spine flat and extend tailbone
Lift navel center, engage abdominal wall
Draw shoulder blades back and down the spine
Gaze slightly in front of fingers to keep the neck neutral

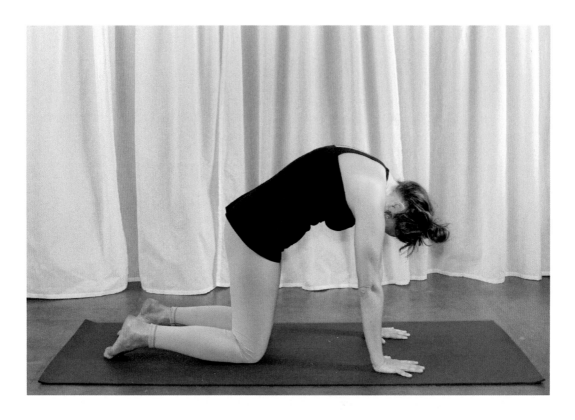

Cat (Marjaryasana)

Stack hips over knees
Spiral the thighs toward the midline of the body
Align wrist, elbows and shoulders
Press palms flat
Spread shoulder blades, engage the abdominal wall
Draw tailbone down
Arch the back
Gaze toward thumbs or navel center

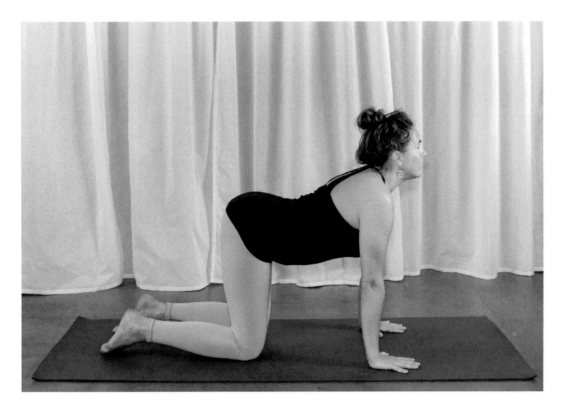

Cow (Bitilasana)

Stack hips over knees
Spiral the thighs toward the midline of the body
Align wrist, elbows and shoulders
Press palms flat
Inhale, lift tailbone up and broaden the chest reverse the arch
    of the spine
Draw shoulder blades back and down the spine
Gaze forward or slightly up to keep the neck neutral

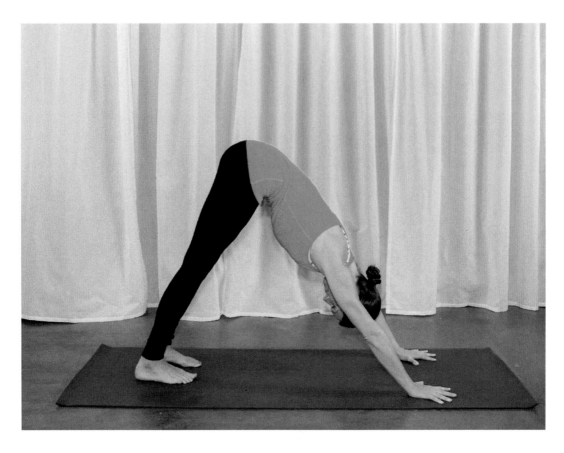

Downward Facing Dog (Adho Mukha Svanasana)

Place feet hip width distance apart, parallel to the sides
       of the mat
Spiral inner thighs in and lift up
Press palms flat on the mat, hands shoulder width distance apart
Rotate inside of the elbow crease toward the front of the mat
Externally rotate biceps
Spread the shoulders back and up, broaden the chest
Lift navel center in and up, engage the abdominal wall
Lengthen the tailbone
Gaze toward the navel or thighs to keep the neck neutral

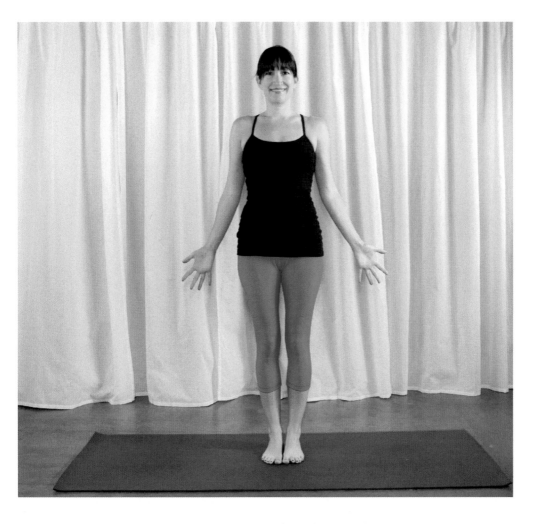

Mountain (Tadasana)

Bring big toes together, feet parallel to the sides of the mat
Ground down through all four corners of the feet
Spiral inner thighs in and lift up
Spread sits bones apart, lengthen tailbone towards the heels
Lift the navel center in and up, engage the abdominal wall
Palms face forward and spread the fingers actively
Draw shoulders back down the spine
Gaze remains neutral to keep the head balanced and neck long

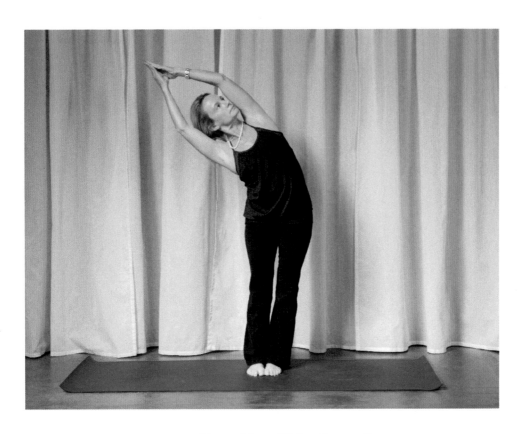

Standing Side-Stretch

Bring big toes to touch, feet parallel to the sides of the mat
Ground down through all four corners of the feet
Spiral and lift thighs inward toward center line of the body
Draw the navel center in and up to engage the abdominal wall
Maintain lift through the sides of the rib cage
Extend reaching arm up and over the shoulder to lengthen the
        side body from hip to armpit, activate lower arm
Square shoulders to front of mat
Gaze forward, up or down to support and balance the head
Tighten gluts to support the length of the extended side body

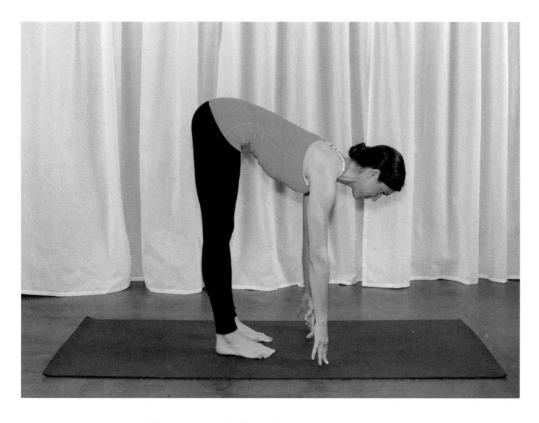

Half Way Lift (Ardha Uttanasana)

Bring big toes together, feet parallel to sides of mat
Ground down through the four corners of both feet
Spiral thighs inward and lift up
Spread sits bone apart, lengthen the tailbone
Lift the navel center in and up, keep the abdominals engaged
Hinge at the hips
Place fingertips on the floor or shins, or palms to knees
Lift torso away from thighs, flatten the back
Keep side bodies long, soften the knees
Draw shoulders down the spine
Gaze just in front of fingers to keep neck neutral
Straighten the legs to your degree, avoid locking out the knees

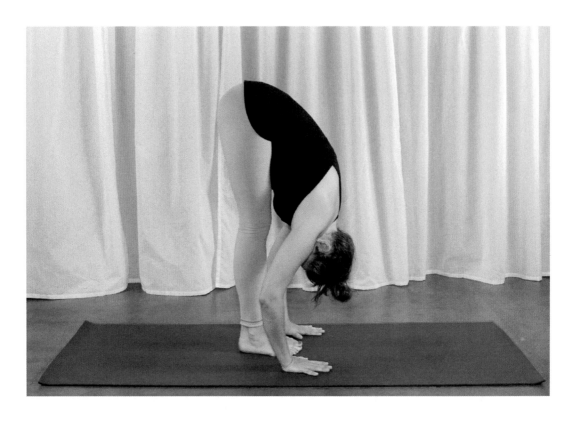

Forward Fold (Uttanasana)

Bring big toes together, feet parallel to sides of mat
Ground down through the four corners of both feet
Spiral and lift thighs inward toward center line of the body
Spread sits bone apart, lengthen the tailbone
Lift the navel center in and up, keep the abdominals engaged
Hinge at the hips and fold forward, keep knees soft
Lift shoulders toward the hips
Place palms or fingertips on the floor or shins, or palms to knees
Straighten the legs to your degree avoid locking out the knees
Gaze to neutral position between shins, knees or navel

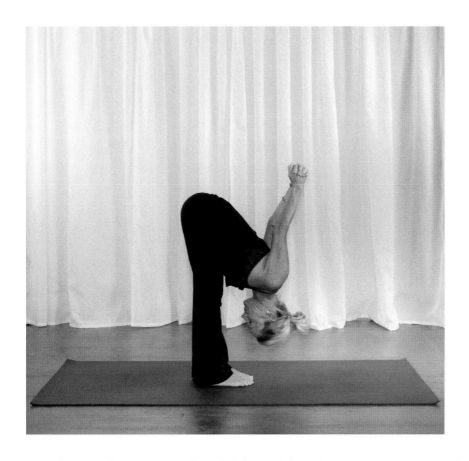

Bound Hands Forward Fold (Badda Hasta Uttanasana)

Place feet parallel to sides of mat and together
Bend the knees slightly to protect the lower back
Spiral and lift inner thighs to the midline of body
Spread the sits bones wide
Lengthen the tailbone
Hinge the torso forward from the hip crease
Engage the abdominal wall
Gaze to the knees to lengthen the back of the neck
Draw shoulder blades together and lift toward the hips
Bend elbows and straighten arms several times to loosen
        tightness in shoulders and neck

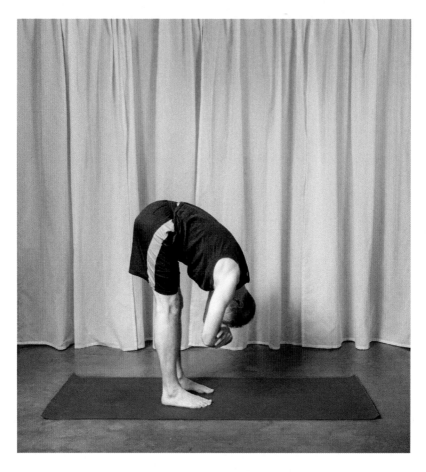

Rag Doll (Uttanasana)

Align feet parallel to sides of mat, hip width distance apart
Bend the knees slightly to protect the lower back
Spiral and lift thighs inward to the midline of the body
Spread the sits bones wide
Lengthen the tailbone
Hinge the torso forward from the hip crease
Engage the abdominal wall
Gaze to the knees to keep neck long
Lift the shoulder blades together and toward the hips
Opposite hands to elbows, activate arms

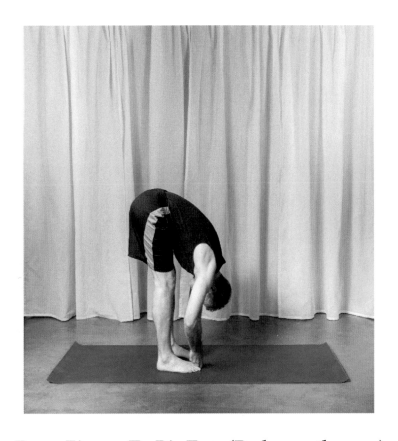

Peace Fingers To Big Toes (Padangusthasana)

Align feet parallel to sides of mat, hip width distance apart
Slightly bend the knees to protect the lower back
Spiral inner thighs to the midline of the body and lift upward
Spread the sits bones wide, lengthen the tailbone
Hinge the torso forward from the hip crease not the waist
Engage the abdominal wall
Gaze to the knees to keep the neck long
Lift the shoulder blades together and toward the hips
Hook peace fingers (first and second fingers) between the first
and second toes
Press down with feet and pull up with arms
Lengthen the side bodies and bend elbows to deepen the pose

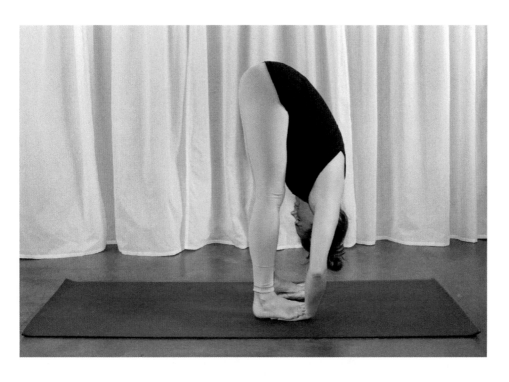

<u>Hand Under Foot (Pada Hastasana)</u>

Align feet parallel to sides of mat, hip width distance apart
Bend knees slightly to protect the lower back
Spiral and lift inner thighs to the midline of the body
Spread the sits bones wide
Lengthen the tailbone
Hinge the torso forward from the hip crease not the waist
Engage the abdominal wall
Gaze to the knees to keep the neck long
Lift the shoulder blades together and toward the hips
Press toes to the wrist creases, shift body weight forward
Bend the elbows and lengthen the spine
Broaden the chest
Lengthen the side bodies and bend elbows to deepen the pose

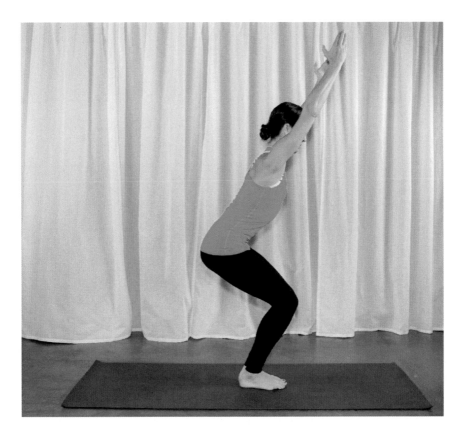

Chair (Utkatasana)

Bring feet together and parallel with the edge of the mat
Touch big toes together, press feet into the ground
Bend knees, spiral inner thighs inward, shift weight back
Lengthen tailbone keep the pelvis neutral
Engage the abdominal wall
Elongate the spine, broaden chest
Draw shoulder blades back and down the spine
Extend and straighten arms upward shoulder width
        distance apart
Turn pinky fingers toward centerline
Draw shoulders down away from ears
Gaze remains neutral to keep the head balanced and neck long

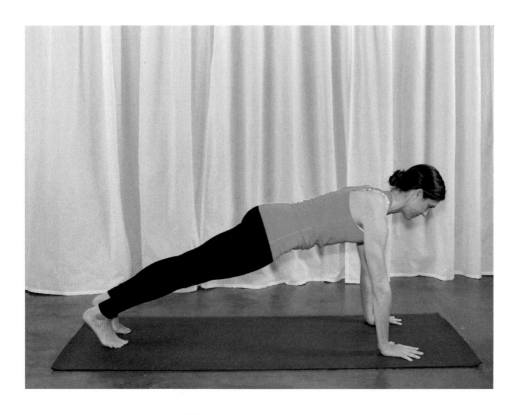

Plank (Dandasana)

Place feet parallel and hips width distance apart
Press down with the balls of the feet and back with the heels
Roll inner thighs in and up
Engage abdominal wall
Spread fingers evenly, flatten palms
Press palms shoulder width distance apart
Stack wrist, elbows and shoulders in alignment
Align hips lower than the shoulders, lift the navel in and up
Lengthen the tailbone
Draw shoulder blades back and down the spine
Broaden the chest
Gaze about 5-6 inches in front of the hands to keep neck neutral
Lower knees to modify

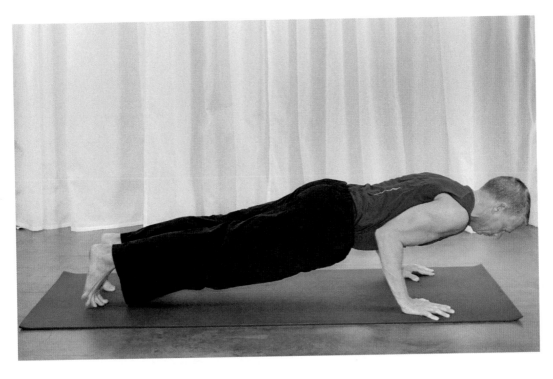

Low Push-Up (Chaturanga Dandasana)

Place feet parallel and hip width distance apart on the
      balls of the feet or toes, press heels back

Roll inner thighs in and up

Extend tailbone and engage the abdominal wall

Level hips with shoulders

Place hands shoulder width distance apart

Press palms flat with fingers spread evenly

Bend elbows up to 90° with the shoulders in line
      with the elbows

Draw elbows in toward the rib cage

Gaze 6-8 inches in front of the finger tips

Keep the neck and head in a neutral position

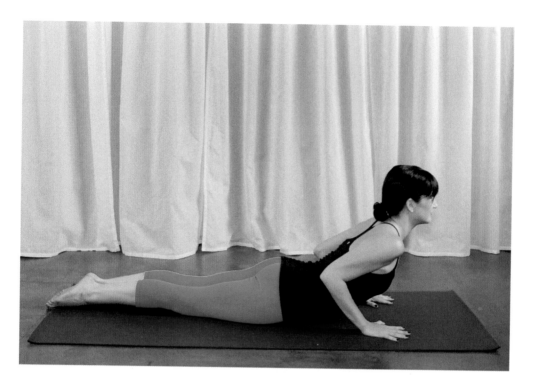

Cobra (Bhujangasana)

Press tops of feet lightly into the mat, bring big toes to touch
Spiral thighs in and up
Press hip bones into the mat, keep the pelvis neutral
Lengthen the tailbone, soften the buttocks
Engage the abdominal wall
Align palms with the chest
Press palms flat lightly into the mat, spread fingers
Bend elbows back to about 45°, hug arms close to the side body
Lift chest and squeeze the shoulder blades
     up, back and down the spine
Keep gaze neutral
Allow the neck to remain a natural extension of the spine

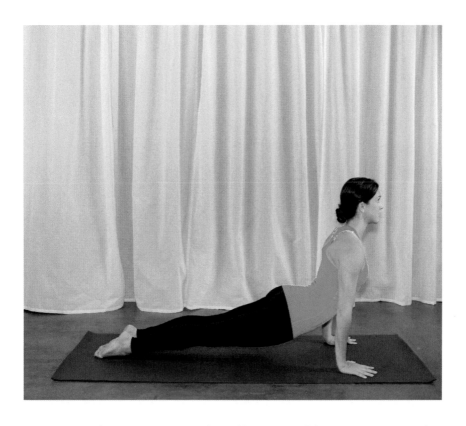

Upward Facing Dog (Urdhva Mukha Svanasana)

Place feet hips width distance apart
    with heels toward the ceiling
Press the tops of the feet/toes into the mat to lift the thighs
Spiral inner thighs in and up
Extend the tailbone, lift the navel center in and up
    to protect the lower back
Place hands shoulder width distance apart, press palms flat,
    spread fingers (stack wrists, elbows, and shoulders)
Lower shoulders away from the ears, spread the collar bones
    apart to broaden the chest
Gaze forward to keep the neck and head in a neutral position
Balance head between the shoulders

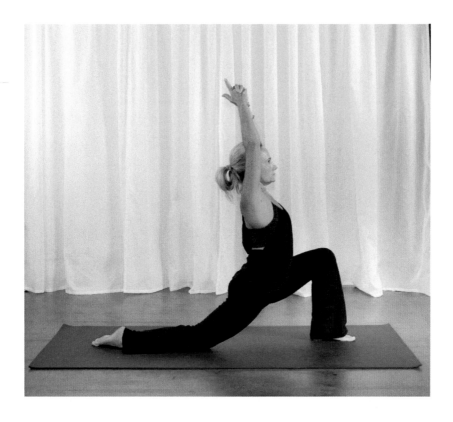

<u>Monkey (Kapyasana)</u>

Align feet hip width distance apart
Stack forward knee over front ankle
Balance evenly between the top of the back foot and knee,
    and the front foot and knee
Spiral inner thighs to the midline of the body, level hips
Lengthen tailbone
Engage and lift abdominals
Lift and broaden the chest
Squeeze shoulder blades together, draw shoulders down
    away from ears
Lengthen and activate arms over the head
Align biceps beside the ears
Press palms together
Gaze either neutral or slightly upward

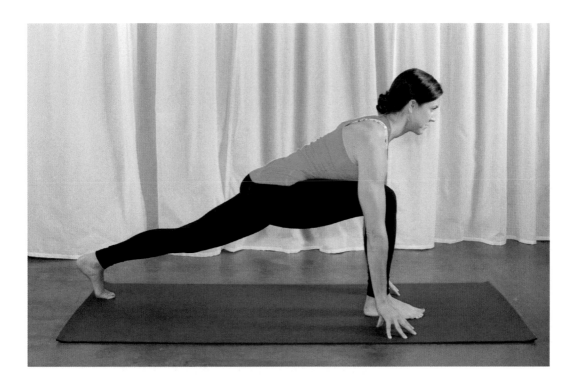

Runner's Lunge

Align feet hip width distance apart
Stack forward knee over front ankle
Press into the ball of the back foot to keep back leg
      long and stable
Spiral and lift inner thighs to the midline of the body
Lengthen tailbone
Engage abdominal wall
Draw forward hip back, allow the waistline to remain long
Incline the spine from tailbone to crown of the head
Press lighting into palms or fingertips
Place hands directly under shoulders
Draw shoulders back and down the spine
Gaze toward the top edge of mat to keep the neck neutral

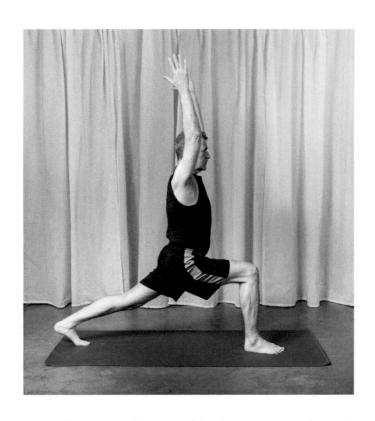

Crescent Lunge (Anjaneyasana)

Align feet hip width distance apart
Stack forward knee over front ankle
Press into the ball of the back foot to keep back leg
    long and stable
Spiral inner thighs to the midline of the body
Lengthen tailbone, engage abdominal wall
Draw forward hip back and level the hips
Extend and activate arms over the shoulders
Stack shoulders over hips, draw shoulders down
Align palms shoulder width apart
Rotate pinky fingers toward the midline
Elongate the spine, balance head between shoulders
Gaze forward or up toward the thumbs

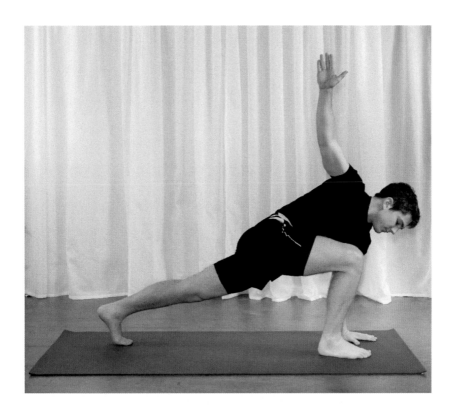

Runner's Lunge Arm Up

Align feet hip width distance apart, stack forward knee over
        front ankle, track knee with front big toe
Press into the ball of the back foot to keep back leg
        long and stable
Balance evenly on the front and back foot
Spiral and lift inner thighs to the midline of the body
Lengthen tailbone, engage abdominals
Draw front hip back, allow the side bodies to remain long
Spiral lifted ribcage upward, elongate the spine
Align upper shoulder over lower shoulder
Place bottom hand to ground, flatten palm or press
        evenly into finger tips
Engage lifted arm, activate the hand
Gaze neutral to keep the neck long and head balanced

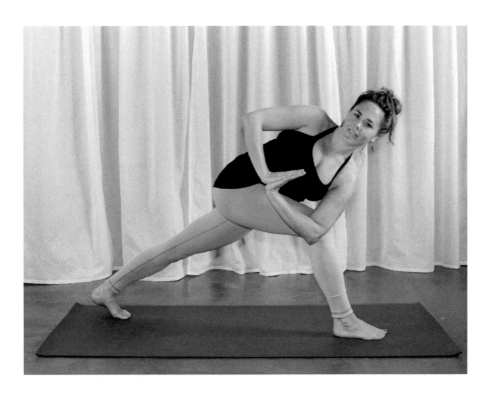

Twisted Crescent Lunge (Parivitta Anjaneysasna)

Align feet hip width distance apart, stack forward knee over
      front ankle, track knee with front big toe
Press into the ball of the back foot to keep back leg
      long and stable
Distribute weight evenly on the front and back foot
Spiral inner thighs to the midline of the body, lengthen tailbone
Engage abdominal wall, level the hips
Draw front hip back, allow the side bodies to remain long
Incline the spine from tailbone to crown of the head
Press triceps to the outer knee or thigh
Align prayer hands to chest center
Stack shoulders, draw shoulder blades down the spine
Gaze is neutral, keep neck stable and head balanced

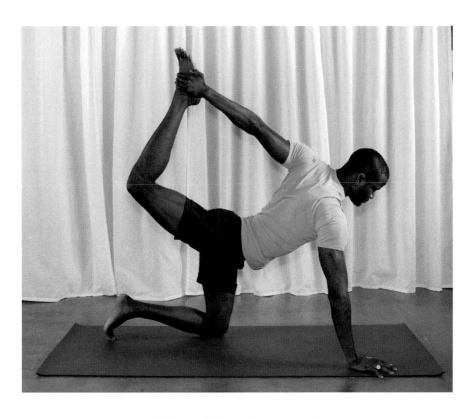

Tiger (Vyaghrasana)

Align standing knee to floor under standing hip
Tuck toes to lessen pressure from the knee
Spiral the inner thighs to the midline
Press grounded palm flat to mat, spread fingers wide
Stack wrist under shoulders, engage arm avoid locking out
     the elbow
Engage abdominal wall, lengthen tailbone
Internally spiral the thigh of the lifted leg
Square hips toward the mat
Bend lifted knee up to a 90°
Extend lifted arm back
Position hand to pinky toe side of foot or ankle
Open lifted shoulder away from the center line
Gaze toward the grounded thumb

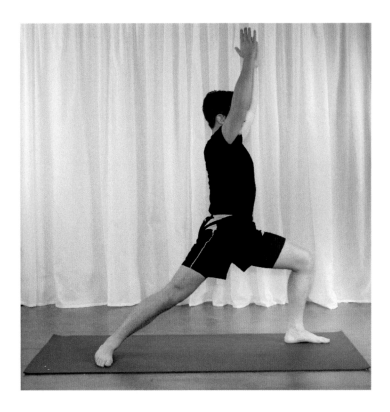

Warrior I (Virabadrasana I)

Angle back foot between 45-90°, press the four corners of
    the back foot down

Straighten back leg, spiral the back thigh to midline

Align feet heel-to-heel or heel-to-arch

Stack front knee directly above or behind front ankle

Direct front toes forward, press into the four corners of the foot

Draw the forward hip back, rotate the back hip towards the
    front of the mat to square the hips

Lengthen the tailbone and engage the abdominal wall

Extend arms over head, pull the arm bones into the shoulder
    sockets, align biceps with ears

Relax shoulders away from ears

Draw shoulder blades down the spine

Gaze remains neutral, keep the neck long

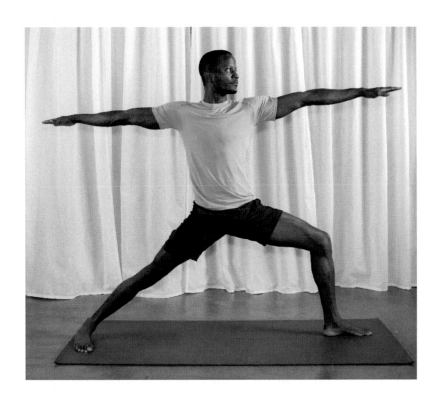

Warrior II (Virabhadrasana II)

Align front and back feet 1 ½ legs length distance apart
Straighten back leg
Press four corners of both feet into the mat
　　*lift the front heel to steer the forward knee outward and
　　place heel back down
Angle back foot 45-90°, lift the arch of foot to support the ankle
Align the front foot heel with the arch of the back foot
Stack front knee over ankle, direct front toes forward
Distribute weight equally between the front and back foot
Rotate and open hips with the torso facing the right side of the
　　mat, align hips under the shoulders
Extend tailbone downward, engage the abdominal wall
Lengthen arms toward opposite ends of the mat in line with
　　shoulders, activate arms, gaze over front index finger

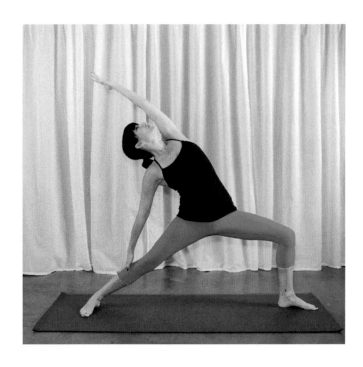

Reverse Warrior (Viparita Virabhadrasana II)

Align front and back feet 1 ½ legs length distance apart
Straighten back leg
Press four corners of both feet into the mat
Angle back foot 45-90°, lift the arch of foot to support the ankle
Align the front foot heel with the arch of the back foot
Stack front knee over ankle, direct front toes forward
Distribute weight equally between the front and back foot
Rotate and open hips with the torso facing the right side of the
     mat, align hips under the shoulders
Extend tailbone downward, engage the abdominal wall
Slide backhand to back thigh, calf or ankle it is a guide, not
     weight bearing
Lengthen through both side bodies (this is not a backbend)
Reach upper arm up and back for a lateral extension
Gaze to the upper thumb, side wall or lower shoulder

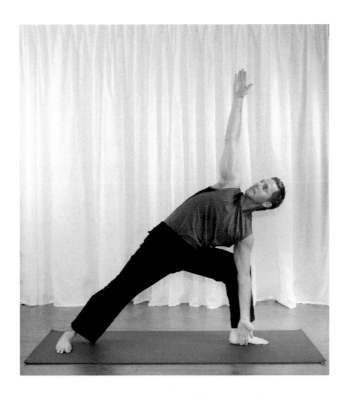

Extended Side Angle (Uthita Parshvakonasana)

Align front and back feet 1 ½ legs length distance apart
Straighten back leg, press four corners of both feet into the mat
Angle back foot 45-90°, lift the arch of foot to support the ankle
Align the front foot heel with the arch of the back foot
Stack front knee over ankle, direct front toes forward
Distribute weight equally between the front and back foot
Rotate and open hips with the torso facing the right side of the
      mat, align hips under the shoulders
Extend tailbone downward, engage the abdominal wall
Stack the shoulders, reach lower arm toward ankle or
      align elbow to thigh
Lengthen the spine, extend top arm above the shoulder
Pull shoulder away from the ear
Gaze to the upper thumb, side wall or lower shoulder

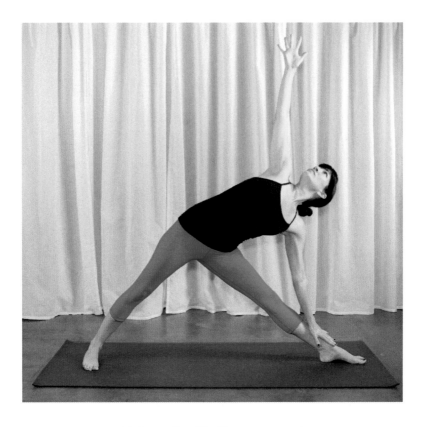

Triangle (Trikonasana)

Place feet about 1 ½ legs distance apart
Anchor back foot at approximately a 90° angle
Press forward foot down, angle toes forward, activate both legs
Hinge forward from hip crease
Draw the left butt cheek up and under
Extend and lengthen through the both sides of the torso
Engage the abdominal wall, lengthen the tailbone
Place forward hand to the shin, reach upper arm toward the sky
Stack shoulders, spread arms wide, broaden chest
Balance the head between the shoulders, neck long, gaze steady

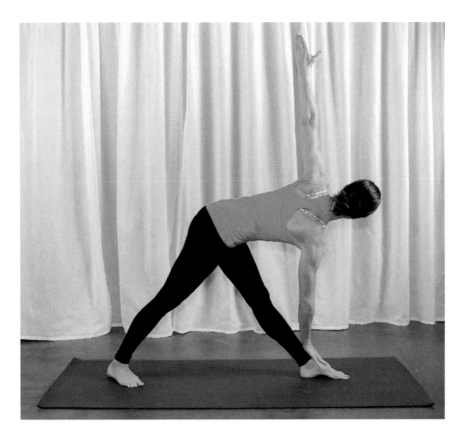

Revolving Triangle (Parivrtta Trikonasana)

Place feet about 1 ½ legs distance apart
Anchor back foot at approximately a 90° angle
Press forward foot down, align toes forward, activate both legs
Adjust stance to feel stable in the legs, keep knees soft
Square the hips towards the front of the mat
Lengthen the tailbone, engage the abdominal wall
Extend the spine, keep side bodies long
Hinge from the hips, reach lower hand to shin, ankle or foot
Draw forward hip back
Revolve rib cage up, open the chest outward
Gaze remains neutral keeping the neck long
Stack shoulders, activate lifted arm

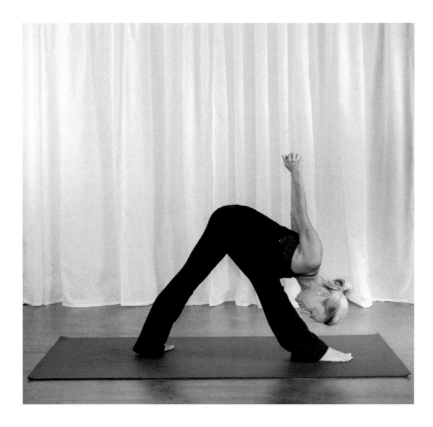

Side Intense Stretch (Parshvottanasana)

Align feet heel-to-heel or heel-to-arch, face front toes forward
    and the back foot at a 90° angle
Adjust stance to feel stable in the feet and legs
Straighten front leg without locking the knee, engage thighs
Square the hips toward the front edge of the mat
Lengthen the tailbone and engage the abdominal wall
Keep the spine long
Align navel center with the front thigh
Broaden the chest, squeeze the shoulder blades together
Lift the arms up and away from the tailbone
Interlace fingers softly to keep from locking the wrists,
    elbows or shoulders
Keep the neck neutral, gaze to the front shin, ankle or big toe

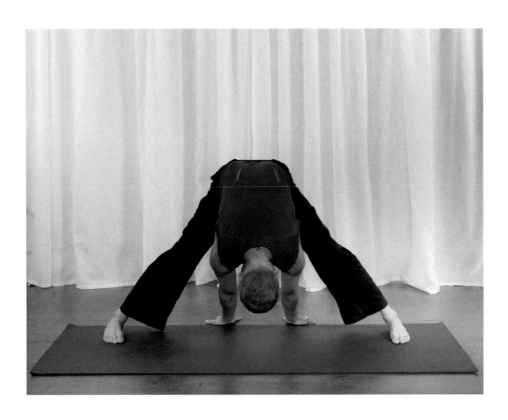

Standing Straddle (Prasarita_Padottanasana)

Alignment feet heel-to-heel, 1 ½ legs length apart
Slightly pigeon toe in, flare heels slightly out
Press down through the outside edges of the feet, lift the arches
Engage the quadriceps and draw upward
Shift body weight forward, allow alignment of the hips over
      ankles, keep knees slightly soft
Hinge from the hip crease, spread sits bones
Extend tailbone upward
Engage abdominal wall
Spread shoulder blades wide
Extend arms between the legs, press palms flat to the floor
Spread fingers away from the face
Gaze between the palms, keep neck long

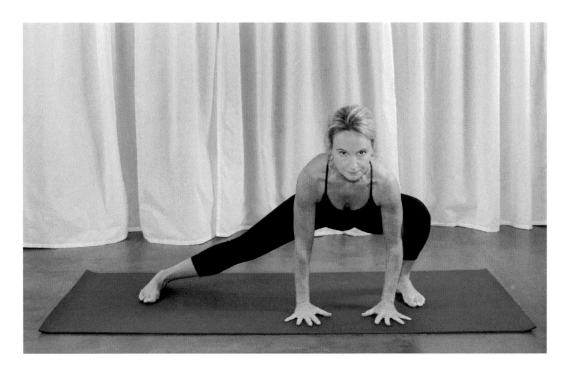

Side Lunge (Skandasana)

Align feet 1 ½ legs length distance apart, parallel to each other
Press outside edge of the extended foot down while lifting
    the arch
Align ankle, knee and hip on extended leg
Press opposite foot flat, align knee over the foot
Engage abdominal wall, lengthen tailbone
Level shoulders, flatten the back
Stack palms under shoulders or prayer hands at heart
Keep side bodies long
Balance head between shoulders, neck remains long
Gaze forward

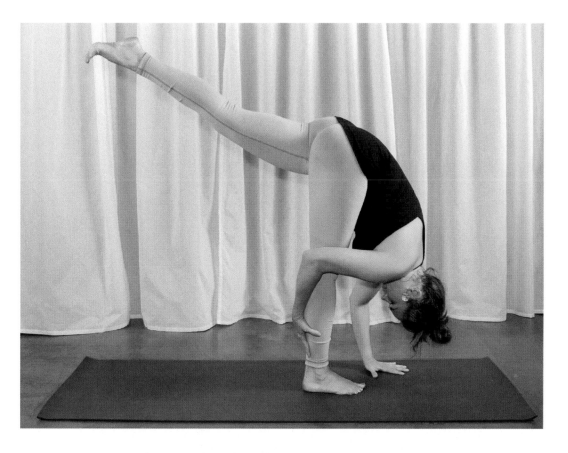

Standing Splits (Urdhva Prasarita Ekapadasana)

Press standing foot parallel to edge of mat with toes facing
    forward, engage leg
Spiral the thighs toward the centerline of the body to keep the
    hips square
Engage lifted leg, flex foot, direct toes toward the ground
Lengthen the spine and the side bodies
Engage abdominal wall to keep from collapsing in the
    standing hip
Place the hands to the floor, ankle or shin
Lift the shoulders away from the ears
Gaze is steady, keep the neck long

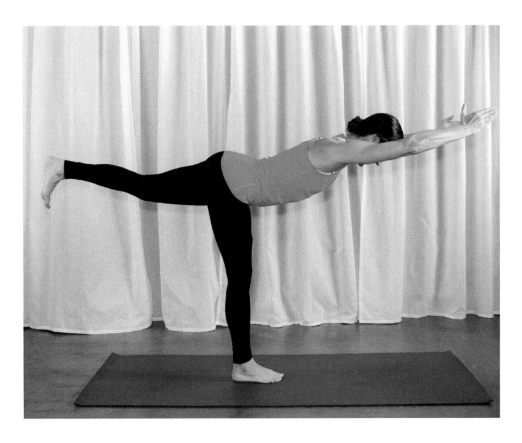

<u>Warrior III (Virabhadrasana III)</u>

Press standing foot parallel to edge of mat with toes facing
    forward, engage leg
Lift back leg to hip height, flex foot, direct toes toward
    the ground
Energize and engage lifted leg, square hips toward the floor
Engage the standing leg to support the hip with energy moving
    upward toward the center of the body.
Initiate core awareness and lengthen the tail bone.
Lengthen the spine, lift the heart slightly to create an updog
    effect with the chest and shoulders
Extend arms toward the front of the mat, align biceps with ears
Spiral triceps toward midline of the body
Draw shoulders back and down the spine

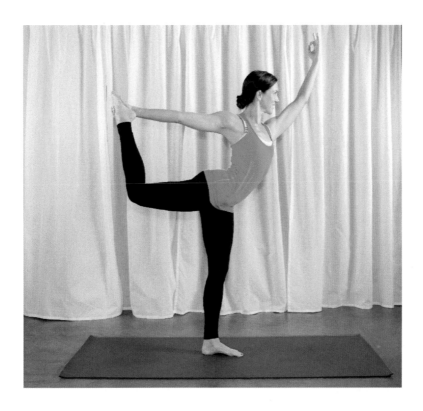

Dancer (Natarajasana)

Press down through the standing foot with toes forward
Lift the thigh muscle up.
Rotate the lifted thigh inward toward the centerline of the body
Square the hips
Engage the abdominal wall, lengthen the tailbone
Spiral right bicep out and away from the body, turn the inside
    of the elbow away from the body
Hold the inner arch of the lifted foot, keep the shoulder open
Lift and press the shin on the lifted leg away from the body
    with toes up
Reach the left arm forward and up
Keep the side body long and broaden the chest
Neck is neutral, gaze is either forward or up

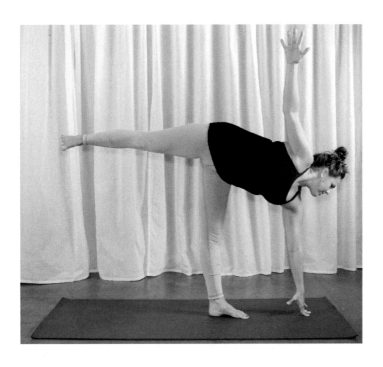

Balancing Half Moon (Ardha Chandrasana)

Press standing foot parallel to edge of mat, align toes forward

Engage the standing leg, soften the knee

Place bottom hand under lower shoulder with the palm flat or
on finger tips

Extend lifted leg to hip height in line with the body, flex foot

Roll top hip open and stack over lower hip

Lengthen and extend both side bodies to prevent the standing
hip from collapsing

Lift up and out of the lower hip so the hip crease
remains slightly open, lengthen the waist line

Activate the entire abdominal wall, broaden the chest

Reach top hand to the sky, stack arm over arm, shoulder
over shoulder.

Gaze up or down, keep the neck long and neutral

Balance the head between the shoulders

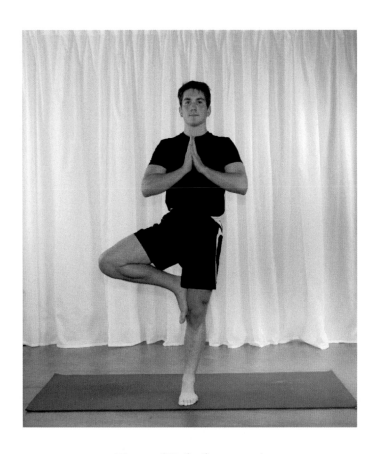

Tree (Vrkshasana)

Press standing foot parallel to the edge of the mat
Direct toes forward, engage the leg
Press lifted foot to the standing ankle, calf or thigh
Open the lifted knee and hip away from the center line
      of the body
Level the hips
Engage the abdominal wall
Lengthen the tail bone toward the standing heel
Straighten the spine, stack the shoulders directly in line
      with the hips
Broaden the chest, press hands to prayer heart center
Balance the head over the shoulders, keep the neck long
Gaze forward

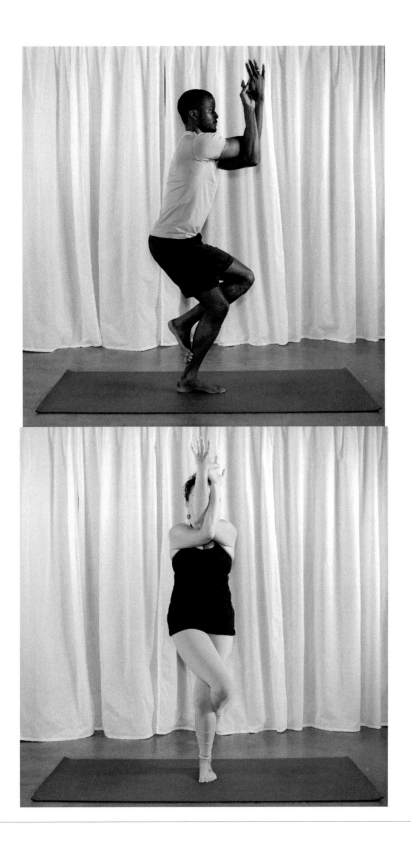

Eagle (Garudasana)

Press down through all four corners of the standing foot
Align toes forward
Bend the supporting left leg slightly, engage the thigh
Cross right leg over the left leg at thigh height
Squeeze or wrap legs together
Wrap the right toes behind the standing left calf if possible
Level hips
Lengthen the tailbone
Engage the abdominal wall
Keep spine upright
Cross right arm under left arm
Bend elbows and wrap to the center line of the torso
Press right finger tips to left palm
Lift elbows to shoulder height
Direct the fingers to the sky
Draw shoulders back and down
Gaze forward

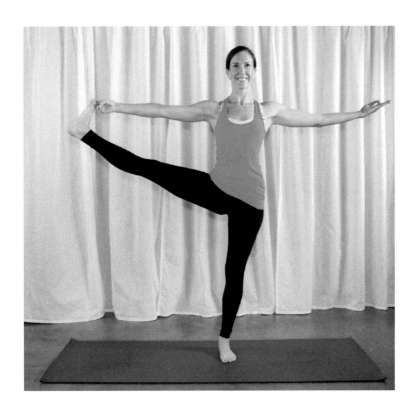

Extended Hand to Big Toe (Utthita Hasta Padangustasana)

Press left foot parallel to the edge of the mat, direct toes
forward, engage the leg
Open right leg/bent knee away from the centerline of the
body at hip height
Support right thigh or toes with right hand or finger tips
Level hips, engage abdominal wall
Keep the side bodies long and the spine straight
Slide shoulder blades back and down the spine
Extend the left arm to shoulder height, keep the arm in
line with the chest
Balance head above the shoulders, keep neck long and neutral
Gaze forward

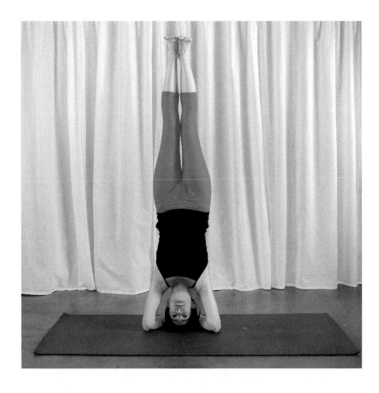

Forearm Head Stand (Shirshasana)

Interlace fingers softly with outer edges of hands and
    press wrists into the mat
Touch crown of the head down lightly to the floor, eyes remain
    still and face soft, lift shoulders away from ears
Press back of the head into the palms, press forearms into the
    ground, form a triangle with elbows and interlaced fingers
Engage the abdominal wall to avoid rounding the upper back
Maintain a long neck
Keep the side bodies long
Stack the hips over the shoulders
Lengthen the tailbone upward
Engage the butt but don't squeeze too tight
Spiral the inner thighs toward the midline, straighten the legs
Flex the toes toward the ground, press heels up

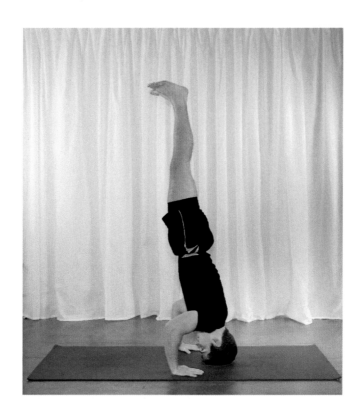

Tripod Head Stand (Salamba-Shirshasana)

Press palms flat on the floor shoulder width distance apart
Spread fingers
Place crown of the head down lightly into the mat so the palms
     of the hands and the crown of the head form a triangle
Soften the face, eyes remain still, lift shoulders away from ears
Bend elbows and drawn inward for stabilization
Stack elbows over the wrist, maintain a long neck
Engage the abdominal wall, keep the side bodies long
Stack the hips over the shoulders, lengthen the tailbone upward
Engage the butt don't squeeze too tight
Spiral the inner thighs toward the midline
Straighten the legs
Flex the toes toward the ground, press heels up

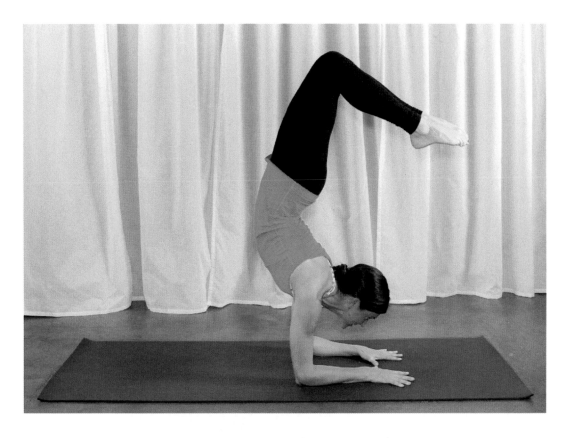

Scorpion (Vrschikasana I)

Press palms and forearms flat, parallel and shoulder width
  distance apart
Spiral inner wrists and forearms in and down
Align shoulders over elbows, engage upper arms
Lift shoulders away from the ears
Gaze between the forearms or elbows
Engage abdominal wall, broaden the chest
Keep side bodies long, lift shoulder blades toward the hips
Squeeze legs together and spiral toward midline of the body
Activate the feet

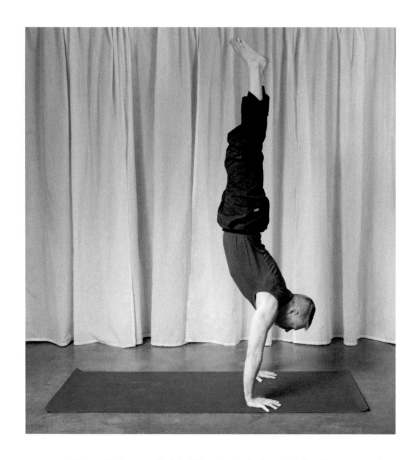

Hand Stand (Adho Mukha Vrkshasana)

Press palms flat and shoulder width distance apart
Spread fingers evenly
Lift the entire body upward as the palms press down
Activate arms, avoid locking out the elbows
Gaze slightly forward of the finger tips
Engage abdominal wall, keep side bodies long
Lift shoulders up toward the hips
Stack hips over shoulders
Spiral thighs toward midline of body
Extend legs to the sky, lengthen the tailbone toward heels
Activate feet

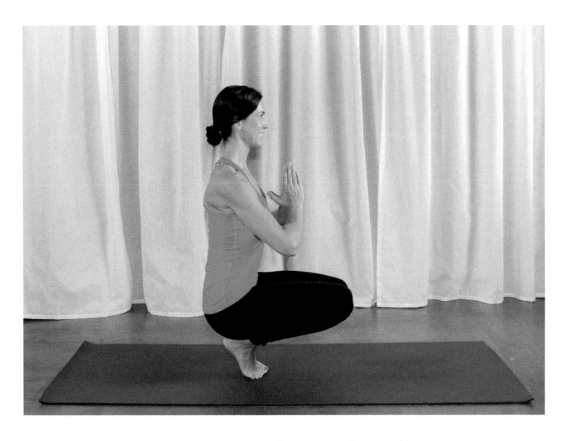

Toe Stand (Prapadasana)

Press all ten toes against the mat, lift heels
Touch big toes together, lock the ankles
Set fingertips to floor to help balance
Squeeze the inner thighs to touch, keep knees together and even
Engage the core muscles, lift the heart
Stack shoulders directly over hips
Draw shoulders back and down the spine
Broaden the chest
Balance head between the shoulders and gaze forward
Palms at heart center

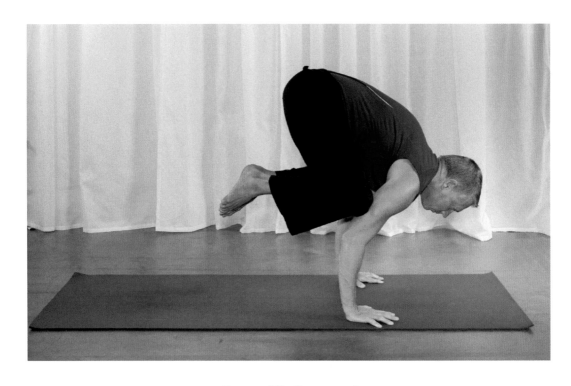

Crow (Bakasana)

Place palms flat on floor, shoulder width distance apart
Align fingers forward, stack and bend elbows over the wrist
Gaze about 6 to 8 inches in front of the hands, avoid looking
   straight down which may cause you to tumble
Lift and press knees to the outside of the triceps on the back of
   the arms
Engage abdominal wall, to create lightness in the lower body
Tuck the tailbone toward the body
Rotate inner thighs inward, lift feet and heels upward toward
   the butt, touch big toes together
Spread shoulder blades across the back, broaden the chest
Balance head between the shoulders

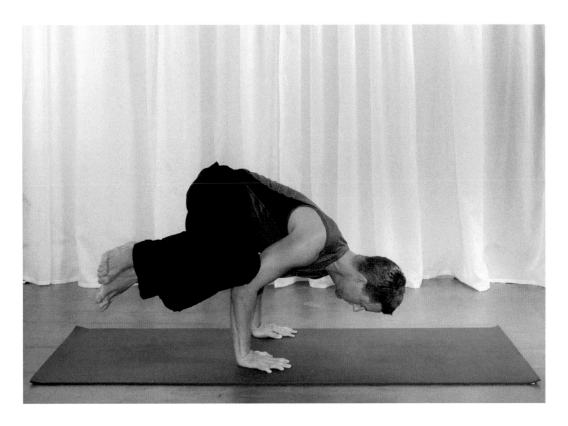

Side Crow (Parsvakonasana)

Place palms flat on floor, shoulder width distance
apart fingers forward
Stack and bend elbows over the wrist
Press and squeeze inner thighs together, lift and align the lower
outer left thigh on the right triceps, avoid the elbow
Lift and press left hip against the left triceps
Engage abdominal wall, extend tailbone
Lengthen the spine, stay long through the side bodies
Broaden the chest, draw should blades toward the spine
Level both shoulders
Balance the head between the shoulders
Gaze directly down not toward the feet

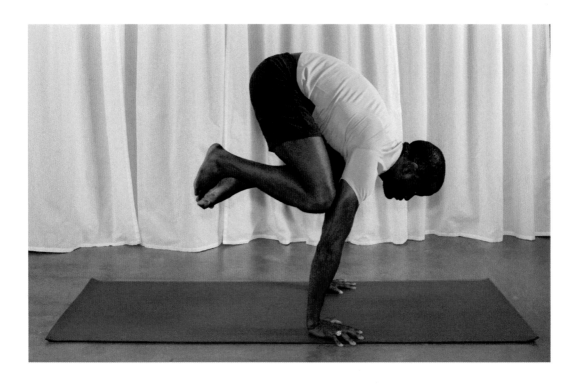

Crane (Bakasana)

Press palms flat on floor shoulder width distance apart,
    straighten arms avoid locking out the elbows
Gaze about 6 to 8 inches in front of the hands, avoid looking
    straight down which may cause you to tumble
Lift and press knees to the triceps or armpits
Engage abdominal wall, to create lightness in the lower body
Draw the tailbone toward the body
Rotate inner thighs inward, lift the feet and heels upward toward
    the butt, cross feet or ankles, or touch big toes together
Spread shoulder blades across the back
Balance head between the shoulders

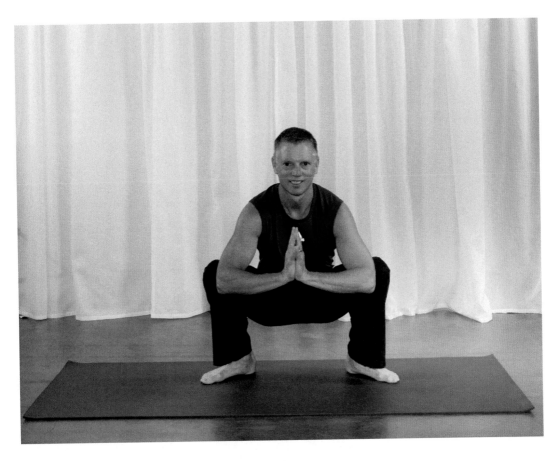

Squat (Malasana)

Place feet slightly wider then hips-width distance apart
Flatten feet as flat as possible
Angle both feet slightly out to open the pelvis
Lower butt toward the heels, engage abdominal wall
Press the triceps against the inner knees or thighs to create a
      greater opening through the groin and hip flexors
Roll shoulders up, back and down
Place hands at prayer heart center
Broaden the chest, keep spine upright and side bodies long
Gaze forward

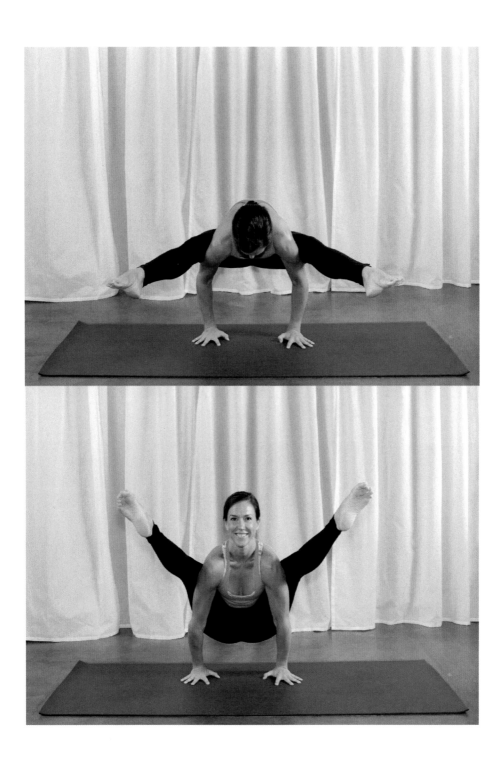

Firefly (Tittibhasana)

Press palms flat on floor, shoulder width distance apart
Straighten arms, avoid locking out the elbows
Engage the abdominal wall, lengthen the tailbone
Place thighs as high as possible on back of arms
Squeeze inner thighs to the outer arms
Press outer arms to inner thighs
Soften the knees to transfer the weight of the pose from
       the feet to hands
Broaden the shoulder blades, hollow out the chest
Lift and extend legs, spread toes, activate the feet
Gaze forward, without tensing the neck

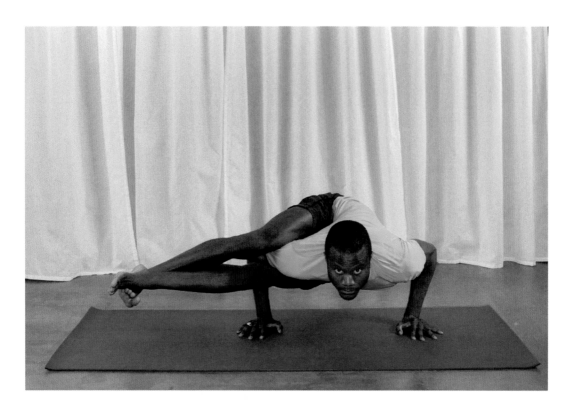

Eight Angle (Astavakrasana)

Press palms flat on floor shoulder width distance apart
Align fingers forward
Bend arms up to 90°, stack elbows over wrist
Engage abdominal wall, keep side bodies long
Lengthen the tailbone
Cross left leg in front of right forearm
Place right leg over the right triceps, cross ankles
Extend legs to the right, squeeze thighs around the right
        upper arm
Balance head between the shoulders
Lift gaze forward

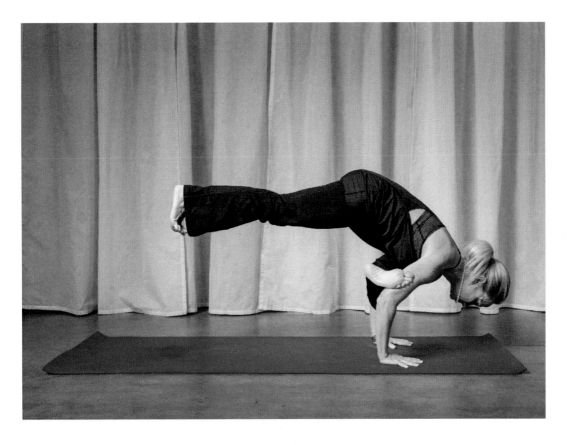

Flying Pigeon (Galavasana)

Press palms flat on floor, shoulder width distance apart
Stack and bend elbows over the wrist
Gaze about 6 to 8 inches in front of the hands, avoid looking
    straight down which may cause you to tumble
Lift and press front shin to both triceps
Hook toes to the outside of the right triceps
Engage extended leg in line with the body, flex foot
Spiral inner thighs
Engage abdominal wall to create lightness in the lower body
Lengthen the tailbone
Spread shoulder blades across the back, broaden the chest
Balance head between the shoulders

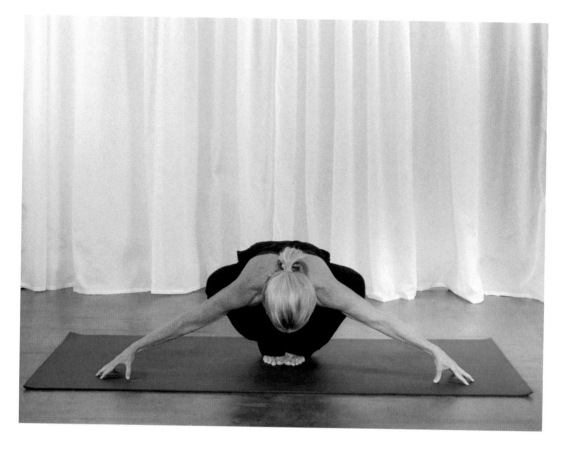

Garland (Malasana)

Bring feet together, touch big toes together, lift heels
Spiral inner thighs inward, spread knees wide
Crease at the hips
Engage abdominal wall
Extend arms in front of the shins
Open chest, extend crown of the head away from the tailbone
Press triceps into the shins or knees
Spread shoulders blades
Draw shoulders down away from the ears
Press palms or finger tips into the mat
Align wrist, elbows and shoulders
Gaze to the toes or navel center

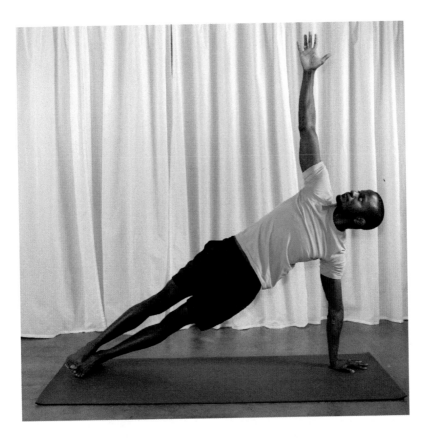

Side Plank (Vasisthasana)

Press lower palm flat, align hand slightly ahead of the shoulder
Activate the arm, soften the elbow, avoid locking out the elbow
Stack the feet, outer edge of the lower foot to the floor
Spiral inner thighs toward the midline of the body
Extend tailbone, stack hips
Engage abdominal wall, keep the side bodies long
Spine ascends from tail to crown of head
Stack shoulders, activate and reach upper arm to sky
Gaze to the floor, neutral or to upper hand
Cultivate a sense of lifting up verses pressing down
Balance the head

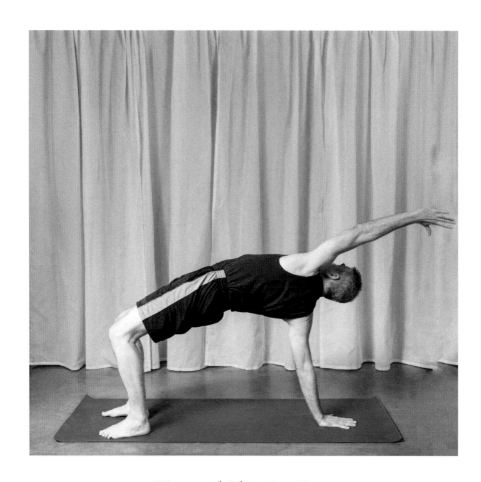

Upward Flipping Dog

Align feet parallel to the edges of the mat at hips width
  distance apart
Stack knees over ankles, spiral inner thighs inward
Lengthen tailbone, engage abdominal wall
Lift hips up and level as possible, engage the butt
Stack shoulder over the wrist, direct finger tips toward the
  top of the mat
Broaden chest, extend lifted arm away from the body
Gaze to lifted thumb or ceiling
Balance head between the shoulders

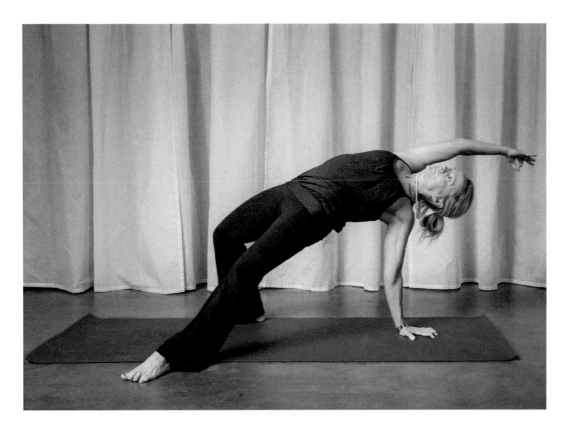

Wild Thing (Camatkarasana)

Press bottom palm flat, slightly ahead of the shoulder
Soften elbow, activate the arm, avoid locking out the elbow
Press onto the ball of the extended foot
Bend opposite knee to support the hip and pelvic area
Engage abdominal wall
Press foot down to lift and level the hips, engage the butt
Spiral inner thighs toward the midline of the body
Lengthen the tailbone
Extend lifted arm away from the body to broaden the chest
Keep the side bodies long
Draw shoulders together and down the spine
Gaze follows lifted thumb

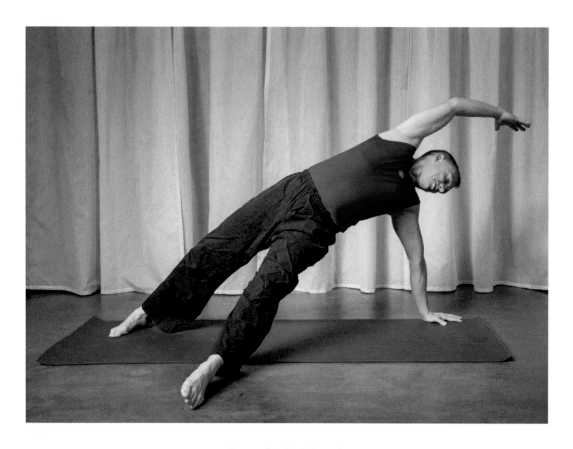

Starfish Plank

Press bottom palm flat, fingers forward
Align hand slightly ahead of the shoulder
Soften elbow, activate the arm, avoid locking out the elbow
Press four corners of the right foot into the floor
Extend left leg perpendicular to the body
Press outside edge of the foot to the mat
Spiral thighs toward the midline of the body
Lengthen the tailbone, lift the hips
Engage abdominal wall, keep the side bodies long
Extend lifted arm away from the body, broaden the chest
Draw shoulder blades together and down the spine
Gaze follows lifted thumb or lower hand

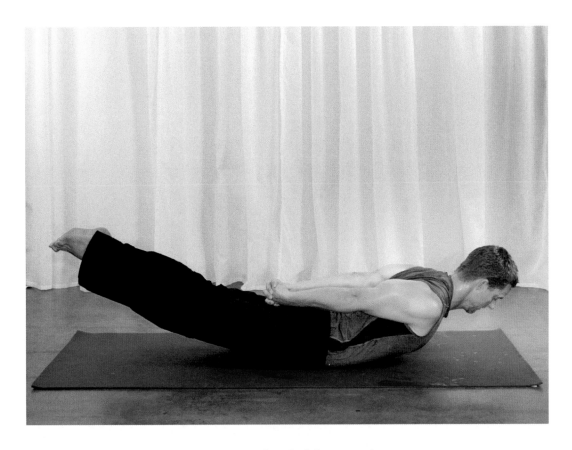

Locust (Salabhasana)

Press the hip bones gently into the mat, keep the pelvis neutral
Bring feet together, touch big toes
Spiral the inner thighs towards the centerline of the body
Lengthen the tailbone, squeeze the butt softly
Interlace fingers at the base of the spine, activate arms
Engage the abdominal wall
Press the hip bones toward to the floor
Lift the legs up off the floor
Lift and broaden chest
Draw shoulder blades up, back and down the spine
Keep side bodies long
Gaze to the floor below the face to keep the neck a natural
        extension of the spine

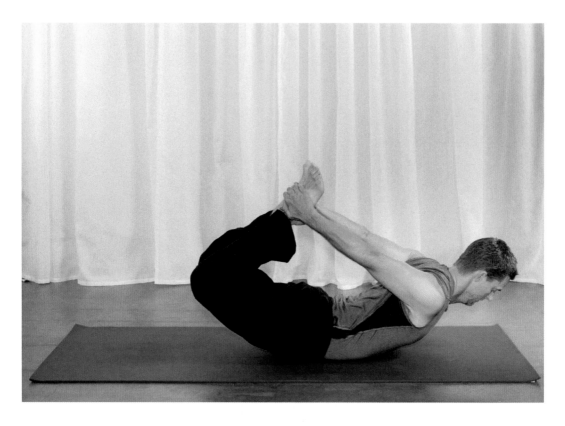

Bow (Dhanurasana)

Press the hip bones softly into the mat, keep the pelvis neutral
Bend and align the knees no wider than hips width distance
Lengthen the tailbone, press the pelvis gently to the floor
Place hands to hold outside edges of the feet
Activate the legs and feet
Spiral the inner thighs, lift the quadriceps up and back
Broaden the chest
Squeeze shoulder blades back and down the spine
Gaze is neutral to keep the neck a natural extension of the spine

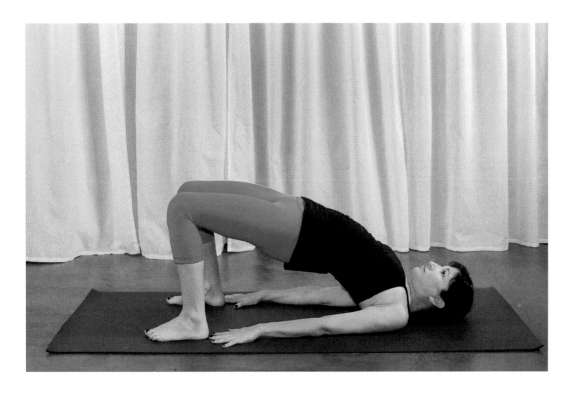

Bridge (Setu Bandha Sarvangasana)

Press the back of skull lightly into the mat, keep the neck supple
Gaze remains still and upward
Lift shoulders up, back and down the spine
Squeeze shoulder blades together
The natural curve of the neck bears no weight
    THIS IS IMPORTANT
Press back of the arms into the earth at shoulder
    width distance apart
Align feet parallel and hips width distance apart
Touch fingertips to heels to assist in placement of feet
Stack knees over the ankles at hips width distance apart
Engage thighs, lift hips and buttocks upward
Extend tailbone
Engage abdominal wall, side bodies remain long
Broaden chest, raise chest to meet the chin

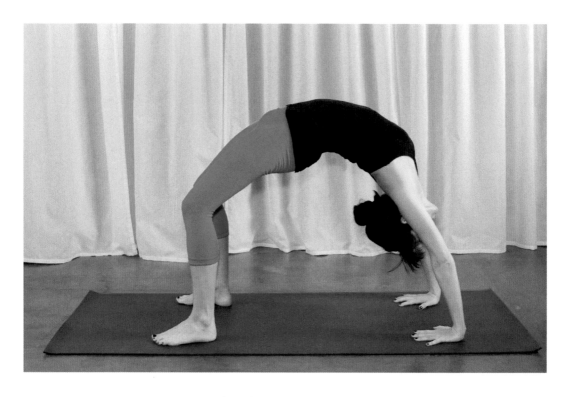

Wheel (Chakrasana)

Align feet parallel and hips width distance apart
Stack and align knees over the ankles at hips width
      distance apart
Engage thighs, lengthen the tailbone
Press palms flat, direct fingers toward the feet
Spread fingers wide
Align hands at least shoulder width distance apart
Extend arms, draw elbows toward centerline
Lift hips and buttocks upward
Draw shoulder blades together and toward the hips
Engage abdominal wall, keep side bodies long
Broaden chest, lift sternum, soften the ribs
Gaze either directly ahead or between the thumbs
Keep neck neutral, soften the face

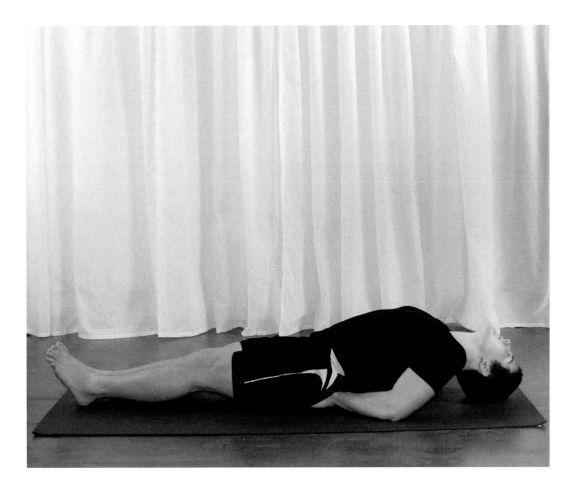

Fish (Sukha Matsyasana)

Bring heels together, spiral inner thighs to the center line
    of the body, extend tailbone
Engage abdominal wall, maintain a long spine
Place palms flat with thumbs under hips
Press wrist and forearms into the mat, squeeze elbows toward
    the side bodies
Lift chest, lift shoulders up back and down the spine
Lift the chin, press crown of the head softly in the mat
Chest and throat remain lifted, soften jaw
Gaze steady

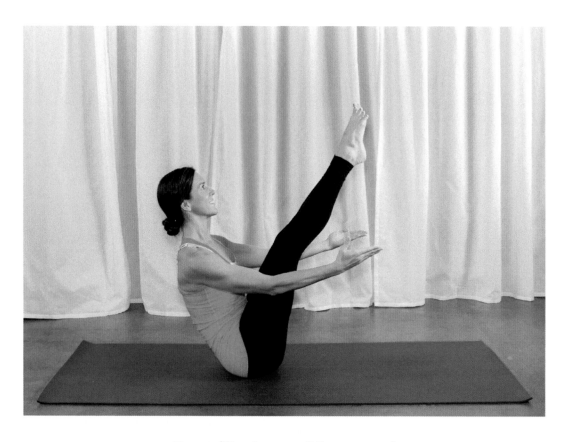

Boat (Paripurna Navasana)

Balance the weight evenly between the tailbone and both
   sits bones
Spiral thighs inward, lift and extend legs
Activate feet
Engage the abdominal wall
Curve lower back slightly
Pull lower ribs in and up
Spread the shoulder blades apart, lower shoulders away
   from the ears
Extend arms forward to shoulder height
Keep neck long, balance the head between the shoulders
Gaze is neutral or slightly lifted

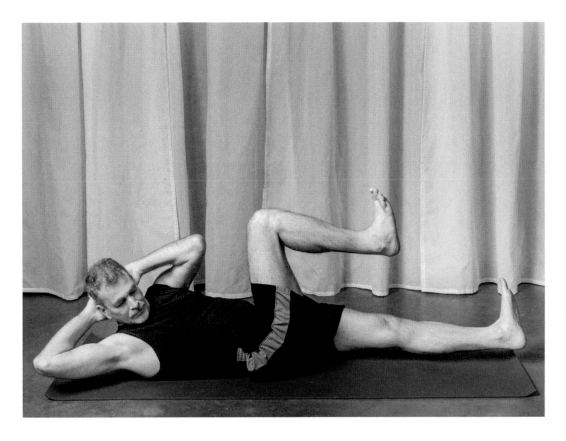

Yogi Bicycle

Extend the left leg forward to the top of the mat, flex the toes
　　toward the face
Spiral inner thighs toward the mid-line of the body
Stack and bend right knee directly over right hip
Flex both feet
Elongate the tailbone, engage the abdominal wall
Interlace the hands at the base of the skull
Extend the elbows wide side-to-side to broaden the chest
Squeeze the shoulder blades back and down the spine
Lift left elbow to right thigh
Repeat same movement to opposite side

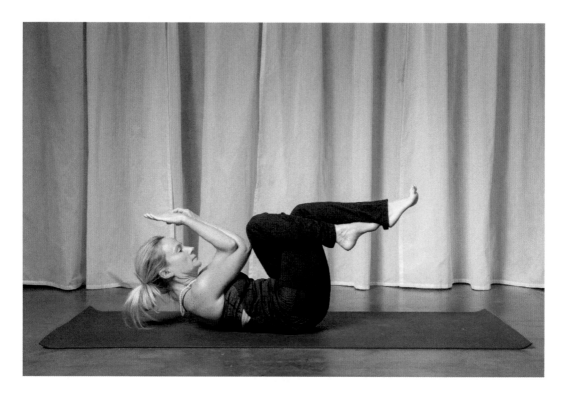

Eagle Abs

Cross and wrap right arm under left arm, bend both elbows
Lift wrist and forearms away from the face
Cross and wrap left leg over the right thigh, bend both knees
Lift shins and feet to parallel with floor
Engage the abdominal wall
On the exhale breath, lift head and elbows and squeeze
    elbows toward the knees
On the inhale breath, lower shoulder blades to the mat while
    lengthening the torso and extending the feet toward the
    top of the mat
Keep all limbs bound
Gaze is neutral, balance head between the shoulders
Repeat with opposite limbs

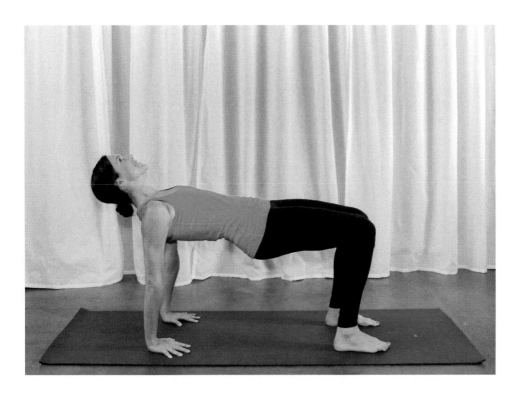

Table Top (Ardha Purvottanasana)

Align feet parallel hips width distance apart, press feet down
Press palms flat with fingers spread, align fingers the same
     direction as the toes
Straighten arms, avoid locking out the elbows
Engage abdominal wall
Draw shoulder blades in toward the spine, broaden the chest
Align knees hips width distance apart
Stack knees over the ankles, spiral inner thighs inward toward
     center line
Align knees, hips and shoulders on the same plane
Lengthen tailbone, soften butt muscles
Balance head between the shoulders, gaze to the sky, neck
     remains long

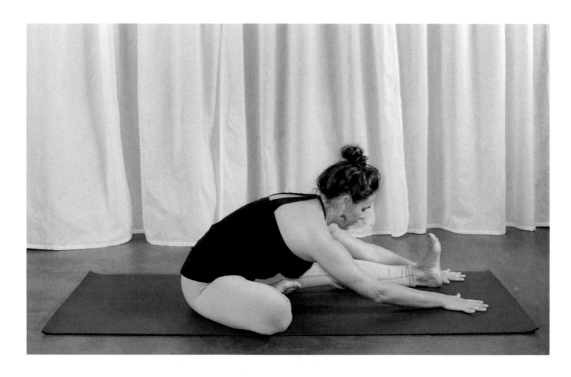

Head-to-Knee (Janu Sirshasana)

Spread and press sitting bones apart and down
Extend left leg to front of mat, align left ankle, knee and hip
Flex left foot
Press right foot to inner left thigh, open knee to the right
Spiral inner thighs toward the midline
Extend tailbone
Hinge forward from the hips, engage abdominal wall
Lengthen spine, keep side bodies long
Broaden chest, lift shoulders up, back and down the spine
Extend and activate arms forward
Bring palms to the ground or left foot
Keep neck long, gaze neutral

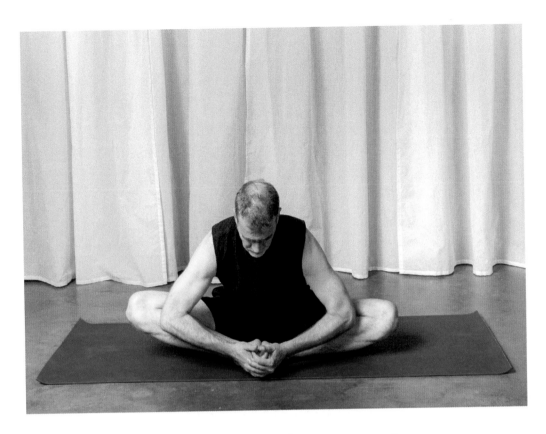

Butterfly (Baddha Konasana)

Press sitting bones to the mat, elongate the spine long
Bring the soles of the feet together
Bend the knees out wide, press the outer edges of the feet
     to the floor
Wrap hands to outer edges of the feet, activate arms and press
     outer arms to calves or thighs
Soften the inner thighs and knees
Lengthen the tail bone
Engage the abdominal wall
Keep the side body long, broaden the chest
Lift the shoulders up, back and down the spine
Keep the neck long and even
Gaze toward the feet

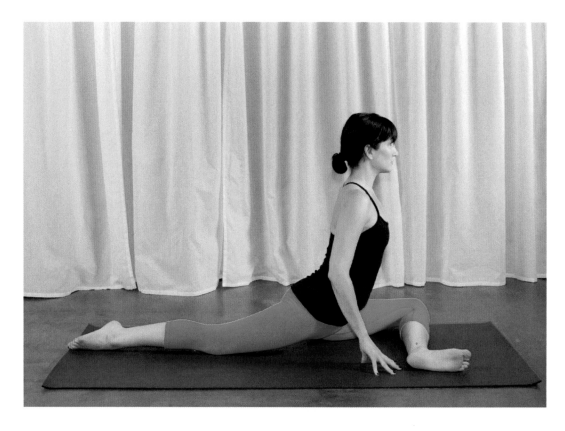

Half Pigeon (Eka Pada Rajakapotasana)

Align left outer thigh and knee parallel to the side of the mat
Bend left knee up to 90° keeping the left foot flexed
Straighten right leg inline with right hip
Press top of foot down or tuck toes
Rotate right hip down, spiral both thighs internally
Lengthen tailbone, engage abdominal wall
Extend spine upright
Draw shoulders back and down, square shoulders to the
      front of the mat
Broaden the chest
Place hands to the mat to balance the torso
Gaze remains neutral

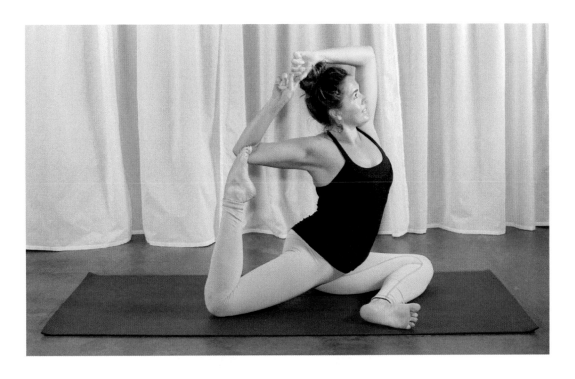

King Pigeon (Raja-Kapotasana)

Align left outer thigh and knee parallel to the side of the mat
Bend left knee up to 90° keeping the left foot flexed
Rotate, right hip down, spiral both thighs internally
Lengthen tailbone, engage abdominal wall
Extend spine upright
Draw shoulders draw back and down, square shoulders toward
      the front of the mat, broaden chest
Bend right knee, roll right hip down towards the floor
Connect right foot to right elbow crease
Extend left arm forward and up, bend elbow
Gaze forward

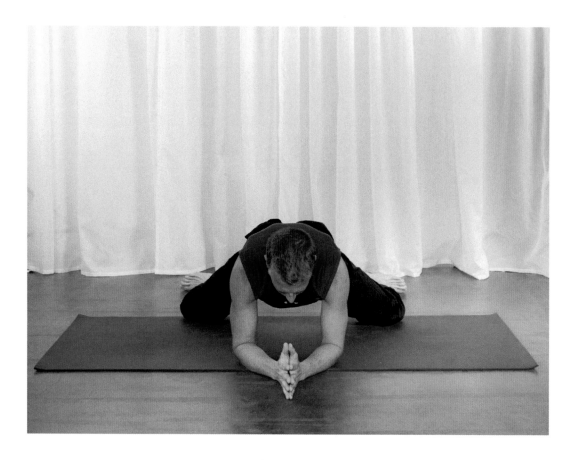

Frog (Bhekasana)

Align heels with ankles, ankles with inner knees, shins parallel
Flex feet, press inner ankles toward the floor
Form a 90° angle with ankles, knees and hips
Spiral inner thighs toward the mat
Engage abdominal wall, lengthen tailbone
Broaden the chest, keep the side bodies long
Stack elbows under the shoulders, level the shoulders
Press forearms down into the mat
Draw shoulders back and down the spine
Soften between the shoulder blades
Gaze remains neutral, keep the neck long
Press palms in prayer or flat to keep the chest open

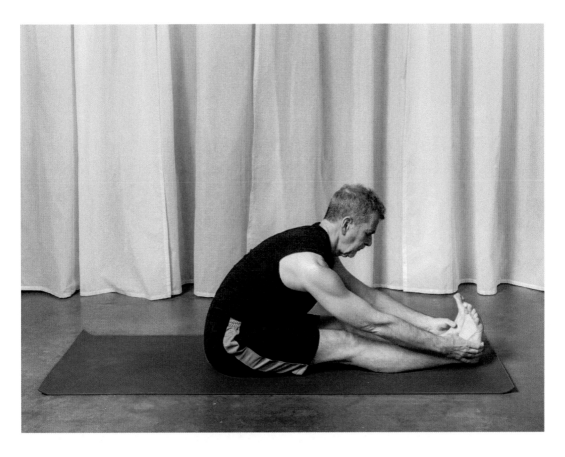

Seated Forward Fold (Paschimottanasana)

Press and spread sits bones down into the mat
Extend legs forward
Lengthen the tailbone, engage abdominal wall
Spiral inner thighs toward centerline of body, soften knees
Activate the feet, flex toes
Lengthen and activate the torso
Hinge at the hips, fold forward toward the toes
Draw shoulders back and down the spine
Reach arms toward the feet, keep side bodies long
Place hands onto shins, ankles or toes
Gaze remains neutral, keep the neck long

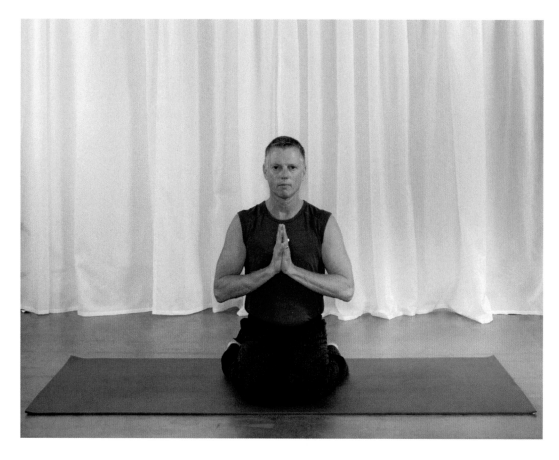

Hero (Virasana)

Press shins, tops of feet and toes into the mat
Spiral inner thighs to center line, align and touch knees together
Roll the calves outward
Set butt between the ankles
Lengthen tailbone down
Press sits bones to block or mat
Level hips, engage abdominal wall
Lengthen the spine upright
Draw shoulders up back and down the spine
Press hands into prayer, broaden the chest
Balance head between shoulders, gaze neutral, keep neck long

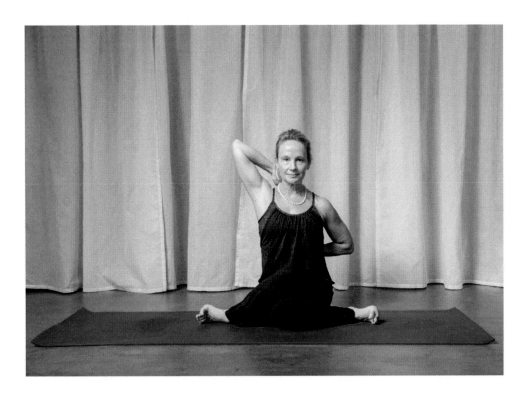

Cowface (Gomukhasana)

Press and spread sits bones into the mat
Cross left thigh over right thigh, bend knees, draw heels toward
the hips
Flex feet to protect the knees, spiral inner thighs toward midline
Level hips, extend tailbone downward, lift abdominal wall
Lengthen the spine
Lift right arm, bend elbow, place hand between the shoulder
blades, press palm between shoulders
Neck remains neutral, balance head between shoulders
Bend left arm at the elbows, reach left palm up the back
Open left palm to touch right fingers, broaden the chest
Keep side bodies remain long, level shoulders
Gaze forward

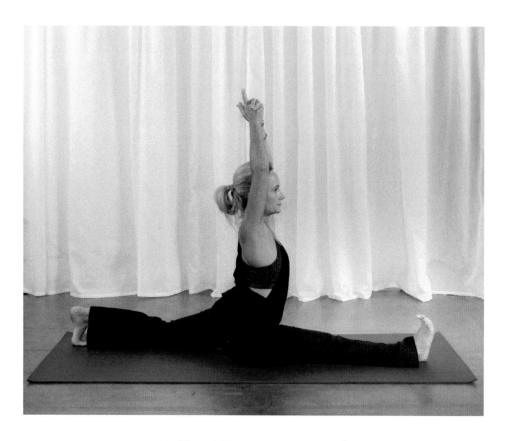

Splits (Hanumanasana)

Press feet to opposite ends of the mats

Press back toes into the mat

Flex forward toes toward the body, knee joints remain soft avoid
    locking out the knee joint

Spiral inner thighs toward midline, press right sits bone to the
    mat, lengthen tailbone, draw left hip forward and down

Level hips to your degree

Engage abdominal wall, lift lower ribs in and up

Extend spine upright, broaden chest

Draw shoulders back and down

Balance head between the biceps, press palms

Align arms over shoulders

Gaze neutral, keep neck long

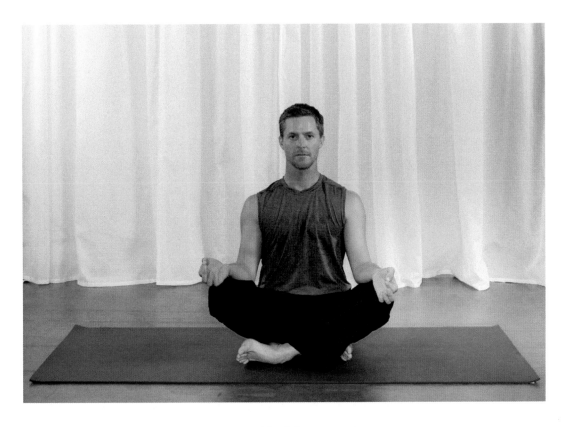

Easy (Sukhasana)

Press and spread sits bones down to the mat
Lengthen the tailbone
Cross ankles, press outside edges or tops of the feet lightly
     into the mat
Allow a comfortable gap between the heels and sits bones
Soften knees out and down
Slightly rotate the thighs inward to stabilize the hips
Engage abdominal wall, keep side bodies long
Lengthen the spine
Draw shoulders down and away from the ears
Gaze neutral, balance head between the shoulders
Rest palms or back of hands on the tops of the thighs

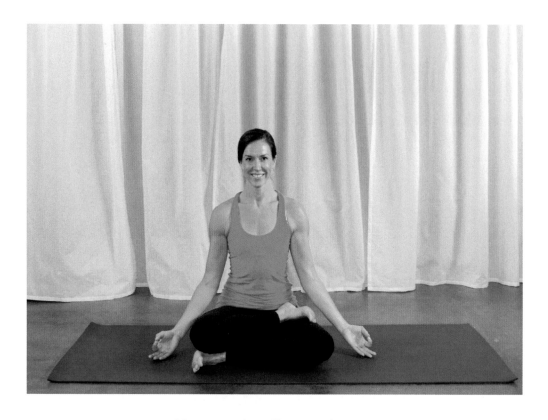

Half Lotus (Ardha Padmasana)

Press and spread sits bones down to the mat
Press top edge of left foot down into the mat
Place right foot to the left hip crease, face sole of the foot up
Soften knees, spiral inner thighs in slightly
Level hips, lengthen tailbone, engage abdominal wall
Keep spine upright
Draw shoulders down and away from the ears
Broaden the chest
Extend and activate arms outward, touch thumbs and
      first fingers, open palms
Balance head between the shoulders, keep neck long
Gaze forward or to the tip of the nose

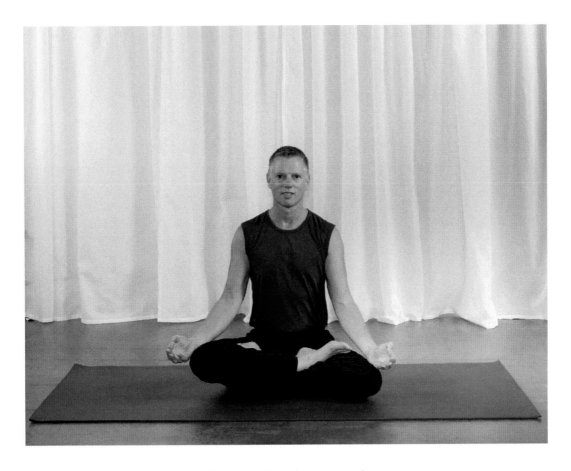

Lotus (Padmasana)

Spread and press sits bones down to the mat
Place left foot to right hip crease, sole of the foot faces up
Place right foot to the left hip crease, sole of the foot faces up
Soften knees, spiral inner thighs in slightly
Level hips, lengthen tailbone, engage abdominal wall
Keep spine upright
Draw shoulders down and away from the ears
Broaden the chest
Extend and activate arms outward
Touch thumbs and first fingers, open palms
Balance head between the shoulders, keep neck long
Gaze forward or to the tip of the nose

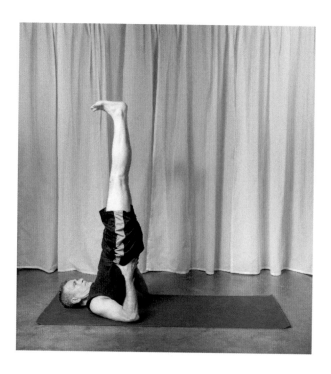

Shoulder Stand (Sarvangasana)

Press back of the skull lightly into the mat, keep neck supple
Gaze still and upward
Draw shoulder blades together, press back of the shoulders
     to the mat
THIS IS IMPORTANT
The natural curve of the neck bears no weight
Press backs of the arms into the mat at shoulder width
     distance apart
Support lower spine with hands
Maintain a long neck, engage the abdominal wall
Avoid rounding the upper back, keep the side bodies long
Stack the hips over the shoulders, lengthen the tailbone upward
Engage the butt avoid squeezing too tight
Spiral the inner thighs toward the midline
Straighten the legs
Flex the feet, keep heels together

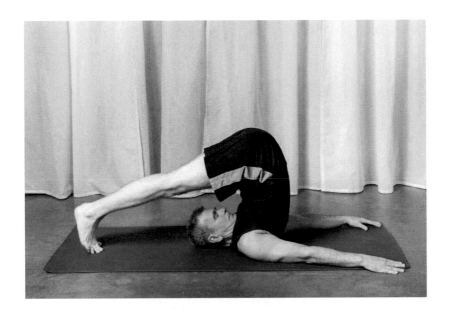

Plough (Halasana)

Press back of the skull lightly into the mat, keep neck supple
Gaze still and upward
Draw shoulder blades together, press back of the shoulders
    to the mat
THIS IS IMPORTANT
The natural curve of the neck bears no weight
Press backs of the arms into the mat at shoulder width
    distance apart
Extend arms long, press palms flat
Maintain a long neck, engage the abdominal wall
Avoid rounding the upper back, keep the side bodies long
Stack the hips over the shoulders, lengthen the tailbone upward
Engage the butt avoid squeezing too tight
Hinge at the hip crease drawing the legs over the top of the head
Extend the legs, spiral the inner thighs toward the midline
Flex the toes toward the ground, keep heels together

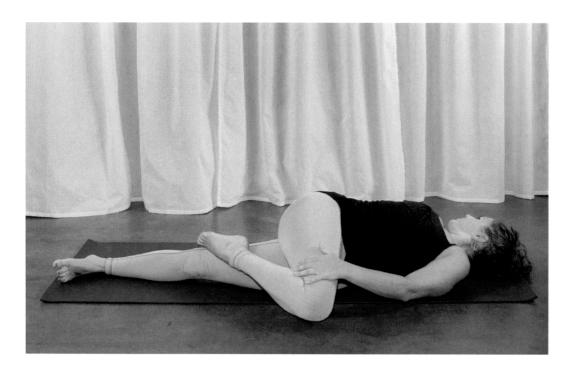

Half Spinal Twist (Ardha Matsyendrasana)

Press back of the head softly into the mat
Keep both shoulders firmly on the ground
Align spine from top of the head to tailbone
Extend right arm in line with the shoulder
Press palm to the floor
Engage abdominal wall
Lengthen tailbone
Rotate right ribcage toward the ceiling
Rotate right knee, thigh and hip to the left
Keep the right shoulder and head on the mat as anchor points
Activate left leg, ankle and foot
Lift head and turn right ear to mat, gaze to the right

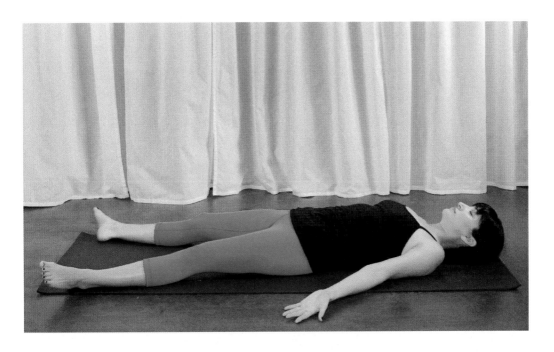

Corpse (Savasana)

Align feet wider than the hips
Open feet away from the midline of the body
Relax the entire body
Keep the spine long with the head balanced between
      the shoulders
Open palms towards the sky to relax the shoulders
Close eyes
Soften jaw
Quiet and ease the breath

Our Special Thanks to Our Yogis

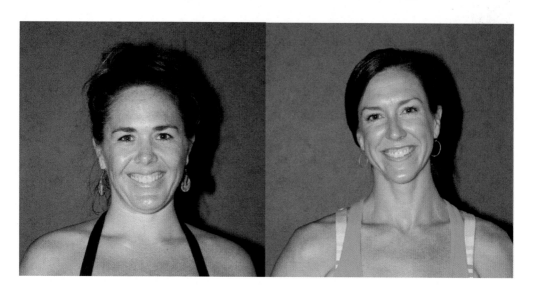

Brennan Edgerton   Ahni Gamboa

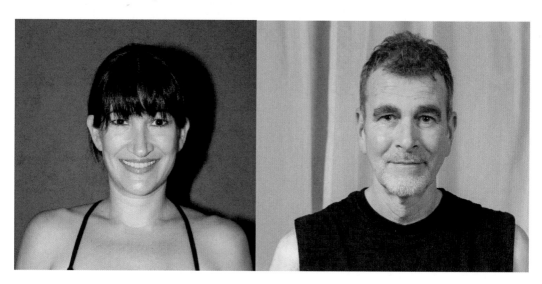

Tessa Todd   John Fynn

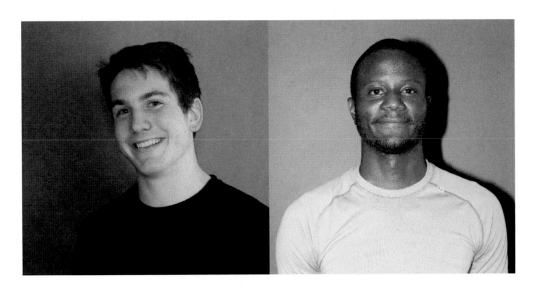

Lucas Burns   **Kemi George**

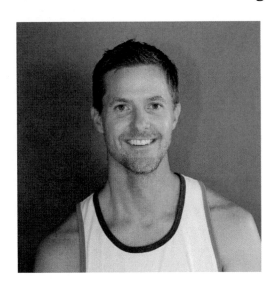

Josh Morgan

English Names Index:

English Names Index: